WHOLE BODY RESET

2 Books in 1:

A PERFECT GUIDE TO LOSING WEIGHT IN YOUR MIDLIFE AND BEYOND

+

THE ANTI-INFLAMMATORY DIET TO DETOXIFY YOUR BODY

100+ Delicious Recipes and Many Delicious Smoothies

Stephanie and Dorothy V. Myller

The Whole Body Reset

© Copyright 2022 All rights reserved.

Written by Stephanie and Dorothy V. Myller

Limited Liability

Please note that the content of this book is based on personal experience and various information sources, and it is only for personal use.

Please note the information contained within this document is for educational and entertainment purposes only and no warranties of any kind are declared or implied.

Readers acknowledge that the author is not engaged in providing medical, dietary, nutritional or professional advice, or physical training. Please consult a doctor, nutritionist or dietician, before attempting any techniques outlined in this book.

Nothing in this book is intended to replace common sense or medical consultation or professional advice and is meant only to inform.

Your particular circumstances may not be suited to the example illustrated in this book; in fact, they likely will not be. You should use the information in this book at your own risk. The reader is responsible for his or her actions.

The information provided herein is stated to be truthful and consistent, in that any liability, in terms of inattention or otherwise, by any usage or abuse of any policies, processes, or directions contained within is the solitary and utter responsibility of the recipient reader.

By reading this book, the reader agrees that under no circumstances is the author responsible for any losses, direct or indirect, which are incurred as a result of the use of the information contained within this document, including, but not limited to, errors, omissions, or inaccuracies.

TABLE OF CONTENTS

BOOK 1: A PERFECT GUIDE TO LOSING WEIGHT IN YOUR MIDLIFE AND BEYOND

Reset Your Metabolism in your Midlife and Beyond with 100+ Recipes and 30 Days Training Plan

Stephanie and Dorothy V. Myller

INTRODUCTION

Dear Reader,

This book will help you achieve the wellness and fitness you desire.

Whether you want to transform your body with the whole body diet, achieve a truly effective detox, or improve your relationship with food....you're about to find all the tools you need, without having to look anywhere else!

Why has the body reset diet succeeded, compared to the multitude of existing diets, in attracting increasing attention and becoming one of the most popular diets at the moment?

The answer is that it works because it is very effective in awakening the metabolism. To have all the benefits promised by this diet, since it involves changes to your eating habits, you need to find in yourself the right motivation to follow it step by step as it was conceived.

The father of this diet is H. Pasternak, a famous trainer who deepened his studies and research in the food field.

I would not define the whole body reset as a diet but more of as a "lifestyle" because 'it's not only based on nutrition but it also takes into consideration another important aspect to be able to lead a healthy life: physical exercise.

The feeding scheme lasts 15 days and is divided into three five day phases.

Every day three meals and 2 snacks are planned, and this applies to all of the 3 phases.

In the **first phase**, that is the first 5 days, the main meals - breakfast, lunch and dinner - are replaced with smoothies.

The **second phase** sees the consumption of a solid low-calorie meal for one of the three main meals. The other two meals will continue to be based on smoothies. It is recommended at this stage to eat two snacks a day

The **third phase** sees the consumption of two solid meals and one meal based on a smoothie. The two meals, as for the previous phase, must have a low intake of calories. This food plan provides an average energy intake of calories between 1,200 and 1,400 per day, therefore you lose weight quickly and you reach the so-called calorie deficit, that is you burn more calories than you ingest.

But you don't just lose weight by emptying your fat mass. You lose body fat by maintaining a toned body.

This is the most important point of this diet and it's obtained thanks to the right intake of healthy proteins and fats contained in the shakes and the meals.

Many scientific studies have been done on the effects of weight loss and calorie deficit. One of the most important ones, which lasted a year, was carried out by a team of experts from the Karolinska Institute in Stockholm in 2012. This study was done on a sample of people who followed a daily diet of 1,200/1,500 calories consisting of two meals and two meal replacement shakes. At a follow-up of one year, an average weight drop of about 8 kg was found.

I am so excited about this diet regimen that I would like to continue to list the many benefits of the body reset diet!

For example, the right importance is given to the fact that foods should be healthy, such as vegetables, whole grains and fresh fruit, and that they should not be processed by the food industry.

In addition, this food plan includes foods rich in fiber.

On the importance of fiber in daily nutrition numerous studies have been done that have shown how diets rich in this nutrient represent an excellent prevention against cardiovascular, metabolic and oncological diseases.

CHAPTER 1

Nutrients Allied to Health and Those to Be Eliminated

In this food plan, protein, fiber and healthy fats cannot be missing from every meal.

Protein

Our body cannot do without this nutrient. Proteins are the building blocks that compose our body: organs, skin appendages, and even DNA are made up of proteins. A lack of proteins can lead to a metabolism slowdown resulting in increased body fat, a weakening of the immune system, poor muscle growth, sarcopenia, depression etc. If you suffer from being overweight it is certainly not for the consumption of proteins but rather for a diet based mainly on carbohydrates and sugars.

Thanks to proteins a hormone that allows us to lose weight more easily, glucagon, is activated in our body.

Here is a list of foods with a good protein content:

- eggs
- fish
- seafood
- low-fat meat
- poultry
- fish and crustaceans
- mixture of whole grains and legumes
- milk and plant based milk
- yogurt and kefir
- cottage and seasoned cheese

Fibers

The fibers contained in carbohydrates are excellent fuel for our body. However it is important to know how to dose carbohydrates because an excess in there consumption leads to increasing blood sugar levels and to accumulating body fat.

So if fibers are taken from the right foods they are an inexhaustible source of health since they promote good intestine functioning and they reduce blood cholesterol levels.

Here is a list of foods with a good fiber content:

- wholegrain bread and pasta among which the one made with spelt flour and oats are recommended
- brown rice
- fruits among which the most recommended are berries, kiwis and oranges
- beans
- vegetables among the most recommended are broccoli, sprouts of brussels, spinach and leafy green vegetables

Healthy fats

The primitive man mainly fed himself on nuts, seeds, fish and animals; therefore, our body is perfectly able to burn fat and as a matter of fact cannot do without it. Among the most important essential fats there is EPA, DHA and Omega 3, contained especially in fish.

Thanks to these essential fats, our body can contrast inflammation, lower cholesterol, enhance our cognitive abilities, improve our eyesight and fight free radicals.

Other fats that you should remember, are the medium chain fatty coconut oil acids. These are easily absorbed by our body so much so that they can provide us with high levels of immediate energy.

They are therefore recommended especially for those who carry out sports.

Speaking of oil, we must not forget the importance of what is called green gold, extra virgin olive oil. This oil plays a vital role in keeping the heart and the entire cardiovascular system healthy. Moreover, it's a valid ally to reduce inflammation due to the high content of vitamin E.

List of foods rich in this nutrient:

- extra virgin olive oil, peanut oil and sesame oil
- coconut oil
- dried fruits such as walnuts and almonds
- seeds like sesame, pumpkin and chia flax
- natural peanut butter without added oils or sugar
- avocado
- olives

Lowering the Consumption of Sugar

More and more scientific studies link overweight and most of man's illnesses with the excessive consumption of sugar.

Excess sugar stimulates the production of a hormone, called insulin, which is activated to reduce blood glucose levels.

Glucose is transported inside the muscle tissues and fat allowing the body to use it as a source of energy, but the excess is accumulated and transformed as a reserve of fat.

The latter is accumulated mainly in the abdominal area for men and on the hips for women.

There is a long series of negative consequences of hyperinsulinemia because of the hormone insulin:

- stimulates the liver to produce an excess of cholesterol
- raises the levels of systemic inflammation of the body
- increases blood sugar levels that promote the onset of diabetes
- increases the levels of water retention and consequently also those of blood pressure

The damage list caused by an excess of sugar consumption would be much longer but what I wrote seems already enough to find the right motivation to put the word "stop" in front of the wrong eating habits and to follow balanced eating regimes just like the one dealt with in this book.

CHAPTER 2

Food Supplements Are Our Allies

To reinforce the beneficial effects of the whole body reset, it may be advisable to supplement it with some food supplements.

Vitamin B-12

Vitamin B-12 is essential for the health of blood and neurological cells as well as for the production of DNA.

Symptoms of B-12 deficiency include fatigue, depressed illness, tingling in the hands and feet, and anemia.

Omega-3 Essential Fatty Acids

Fundamentally, omega-3 essential fatty acids are composed of the various components of cell membranes. They aid the following areas:

- brain functioning and visual health energy
- maintaining good heart health and a good cardio circulatory system

Vitamin C or Ascorbic Acid

Although the food plan of the whole body reset is rich in foods that contain vitamins, can still be important to integrate this vitamin because the cultivation soils today are less fertile than those of the past are and consequently their fruits may not have the high vitamin C concentrations as they used to have.

We are also talking about a vitamin that degrades easily with heat, therefore we are not always able to assimilate it in the right quantities.

It is one of the most important vitamins because it is involved in numerous metabolic and enzymatic processes:

- Strengthens the immune defenses therefore increasing the ability of immune cells to produce antibodies; increasing the body's ability to better resist all diseases.
- It has a detoxifying effect on the body (toxins resulting from smoke or pollution).
- Protects and repairs tissues by affecting collagen production; the latter safeguards the functions of cartilage, bones, skin, capillaries and gums.
- It is antioxidant because it counteracts the negative effects of free radicals or those molecules that push our body towards premature aging
- It is useful in case of anemia because it improves the assimilation of iron which is an important mineral for the production of red blood cells.
- It helps to reduce stress by helping the synthesis of molecules that keep the transmission of Nerve impulses stable; it also regulates the synthesis of the stress hormone.

Vitamin D

Our bodies are only able to synthesize vitamin D when we expose ourselves to the sun.

For those who rarely expose themselves to the sun or only at certain times of the year, it may be useful to integrate this vitamin into their diet.

This vitamin is very important:

- For the correct mineralization of bones and teeth because it helps maintain an optimal level of calico in the blood
- To help keep our kidneys, arteries and body tissues healthy

- To strengthen the system against infections and immune viruses
- To maintain the functionality of the heart and the cardio-circulatory system.

CHAPTER 3

Physical Exercise to Develop Endurance, Tonicity and Strength

You can't expect to get all the benefits from this diet and reset your body without including some movement in your everyday life.

In phase one, it is enough to follow the general health guidelines that recommend walking at least 8000 / 10000 steps every day. 10,000 steps a day means walking at a good pace for about an hour.

Movement accelerates the metabolism, making body burn the accumulated fat in order to produce energy, by sweating, we will eliminate toxins and the cardiovascular system will certainly thank us'!

In phase two you can also spend time on endurance training using weights.

It is not necessary to engage in complicated or overly strenuous workouts.

Good results can also be obtained from a basic workout that stimulates the muscles of a single part of the body for at least 10 minutes a day. The next day you can concentrate on another area of your body with targeted exercises on that area. For example on the first day ten minutes of abs, on the second day you can train your arms and shoulders, on the third day your legs etc.

The key to success is consistency and continuity: better to apply a few minutes a day but every day rather than doing strenuous workouts of more than an hour once a month!

To make this easier, you can find a training plan below that you can start practicing from the second phase of the whole body reset program.

These exercises are bodyweight exercises and you can do them anywhere because all you need is your body and the desire to get in shape.

The first three exercises focus on the lower body

Squat

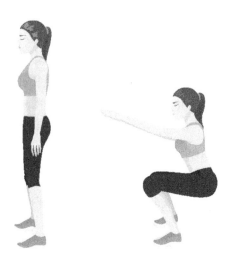

How to do it:

1. You have to place the feet so that they are slightly wider than the shoulders
2. Inhale and bend your knees so that you come down as if you were going to sit down
3. Exhale to rise to the starting position

This exercise is excellent to burn fat, tone and strengthen all the muscles of the lower area of the body and improve the heart's endurance.

It is often recommended to prevent back pain or to eliminate it if already present.

Sink

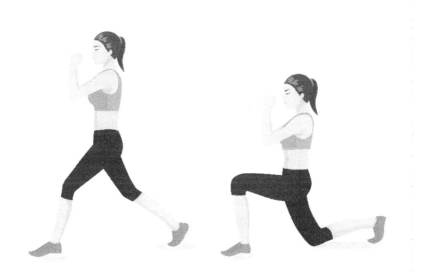

How to do it:

1. You starts from a neutral position
2. Inhale and bring one foot back in lunge until you touch the knee on the ground
3. Exhale and rise to the starting position

Plank

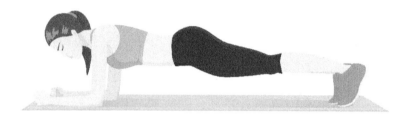

How to do it:

1. You place yourself on the ground leaning with your hands and holding your arms outstretched
2. Shoulders, pelvis and ankles should be aligned to form a straight line
3. To maintain the position you must contract the abdominals and buttocks

This exercise strengthens the abdominal muscles and the whole central part of the body

Side Plank

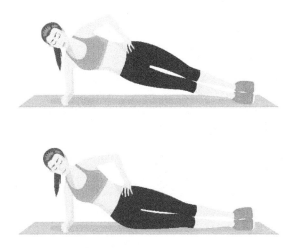

How to do it:

1. You have to position yourself on the ground leaning on a hand while keeping the arm stretched
2. Maintain alignment between shoulders, pelvis and ankles
3. Abdominal and lumbar muscles should be kept contracted

This is also a valid exercise to work the central part of the body called the core.

Stretching Over the Head

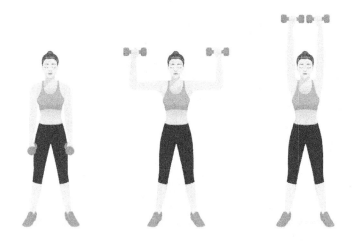

How to do it:

1. Spread your legs apart and align your feet at shoulder level, a two kilo weight is raised by lifting the arms up to shoulder height

2. While inhaling, remain in the position for 30 seconds

3. While exhaling, return the arms to the starting position

This exercise will tone the triceps in the back of your arms.

Lateral Extensions

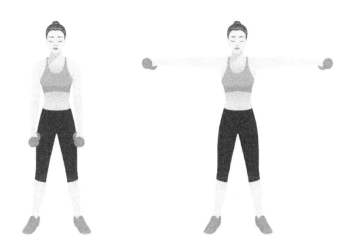

How to do it:

1. Spread your legs apart and align your feet at shoulder level, a two kilo weight is raised by lifting the arms above the head

2. While inhaling, put your hands behind your head

3. While exhaling, return the arms above the head to the starting position

This exercise will tone the triceps in the back of your arms.

Training Program for Weight Loss

This training program is based on a five-day cycle to be repeated.

The program must be done every day where ever you want even at home.

DAY 1

EXERCISE	WORKING TIME	RECOVERY
Running on the spot	4 minutes	
Squat	40 seconds	4 repetitions with a 30 second break at each repetition
Plank	40 seconds	4 repetitions with a 30 second break at each repetition

DAY 2

EXERCISE	WORKING TIME	RECOVERY
Running on the spot	4 minutes	
Squat	40 seconds	4 repetitions with a 30 second break at each repetition
Side Plank	40 seconds	4 repetitions with a 30 second break at each repetition

DAY 3

EXERCISE	WORKING TIME	RECOVERY
Running on the spot	4 minutes	
Pank	40 seconds	4 repetitions with a 30 second break at each repetition
Extensions above the head	40 seconds	4 repetitions with a 30 second break at each repetition

DAY 4

EXERCISE	WORKING TIME	RECOVERY
Running on the spot	4 minutes	
Side Plank	40 seconds	4 repetitions with a 30 second break at each repetition
Extensions above the head	40 seconds	4 repetitions with a 30 second break at each repetition

DAY 5

EXERCISE	WORKING TIME	RECOVERY
Ranking on the spot	4 minutes	
Squat	40 seconds	4 repetitions with a 30 second break at each repetition
Lateral Extensions	40 seconds	4 repetitions with a 30 second break at each repetition

You can use these tables or change the combination of exercises in order to work more on the body parts you prefer to tone. It is however always advisable in the long term to work alternately all parts of the body: upper part, legs and the core part that is, abdominal and lumbar area.

Repeat this program over the 4 weeks of the first month.

From the second month you can increase the time of each exercise by 10 seconds.

By respecting this training plan, alternating it with the fast walk we talked about above, you will visibly improve the form of your body from week to week.

So have **a good workout!**

CONCLUSION

Resetting your body means promoting the concept that instead of eating and taking care of yourself, you can cure and take care of yourself by eating.

But to do this, it is certainly necessary to know and well understand the foods you eat and the effects they have on your health.

We should remember that our body is endowed with a great power: the power to heal and reset itself.

Numerous scientific studies have led to the certainty that an adequate diet and the right exercise can prevent many diseases and in many cases be curative until their total remission.

When you learn how to make food become a "good friend" that helps you feel good and you learn how to do the correct exercises our body will thank you for its newfound health.

If this was what you were looking for, well then, maybe you have found it in this book.

I would love to know your opinion: write a review about this book!

RECIPES

SMOOTHIES: PHASE 1

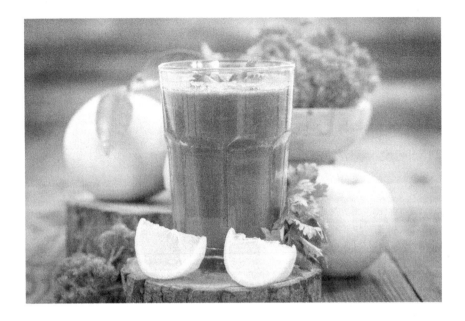

To prepare these smoothies you need to combine the ingredients in a blender and mix until smooth.

At the end of the preparation, the smoothy can be garnished with oil seeds and spices as desired.

Double berry avocado smoothie

INGREDIENTS:

water 1 cup

1/2 cup of raspberries and strawberries

half of a mature avocado

2 cups of fresh spinach

2 tablespoons of hemp seeds

NUTRITION:

Calories: 330

Fat: 24 grams

Carbs: 20 grams

Fiber: 14 grams

Protein: 14 grams

Chocolate Almond Smoothie

INGREDIENTS:

1 cup of almond milk or another vegetable milk

2 tablespoons of creamy peanut butter

1 tablespoon of cocoa powder

1/4 cup of heavy cream

1 cup of ice

NUTRITION:

Calories: 335

Fat: 29 grams

Carbs: 12 grams

Fiber: 5 grams

Protein: 12 grams

Strawberry Zucchini Chia Smoothie

INGREDIENTS:

1 cup (240 ml) of water

1/2 cup of fresh blueberries and raspberries

1 cup of chopped zucchini

3 tablespoons of chia seeds

NUTRITION:

Calories: 210

Fat: 15 grams

Carbs: 18 grams

Fiber: 18 grams

Protein: 10 grams

Bulletproof smoothy

This combination of ingredients boosts metabolism and helps increase energy levels, improve cognitive function, and provide a long lasting sense of satiety.

INGREDIENTS:

300 ml of American coffee

1 tablespoon of MCT oil - you can buy in online stores

1 tablespoon butter ghee - you can buy in online stores

PREPARATION:

Prepare American coffee, diluting it with boiling water.

Add 1 tablespoon of MCT oil and 1 tablespoon of ghee butter.

Pour everything into a blender and blend for 30 to 40 seconds, or until your coffee is creamy.

At your discretion, you can add a pinch of salt or cinnamon powder.

Coconut Strawberry Mint Smoothie

INGREDIENTS:

1/2 cup of coconut milk

1/2 cup of strawberry

2 tablespoons of shredded coconut

6 mint leaves

NUTRITION

Calories: 332

Fat: 28 grams

Carbs: 15 grams

Fiber: 6 grams

Protein: 5 grams

Smoothy detox, with apple, cucumber and ginger

Apple, ginger and cucumber have a high concentration of vitamins and minerals.

INGREDIENTS::

1 green apple

1 cucumber

5 g of grated ginger

200 ml of water

NUTRITION

Calories: 91

Fat: 1 grams

Carbs: 9 grams

Fiber: 8 grams

Protein: 4 grams

Lemon Cucumber Green Smoothie

INGREDIENTS:

1/2 cup of water

1/2 cup of ice

1 cup of sliced cucumber

1 cup of kale

1 tablespoon of lemon or lime juice

2 tablespoons of milled flax seeds

NUTRITION

Calories: 98

Fat: 5 grams

Carbs: 9 grams

Fiber: 6 grams

Protein: 5 grams

Energy Smoothy

INGREDIENTS:

1 Apple

1 Zucchini

125 ml soy milk

150 g Greek yogurt 0% fat

1 tablespoon Peanut Butter

2 nuts

NUTRITION:

Calories: 302

Fat: 24 grams

Carbs: 19 grams

Fiber: 4 grams

Protein: 10 grams

Cinnamon Blueberries Smoothie

INGREDIENTS:

1 cup of unsweetened soy milk

1/2 cup of blueberries

1/2 avocado

1 cup of spinach or kale

2 tablespoons of almond butter

1/8 teaspoon of cinnamon

NUTRITION:

Calories: 296

Fat: 23 grams

Carbs: 18 grams

Fiber: 14 grams

Protein: 16 grams

Strawberries and Cream Smoothie

INGREDIENTS:

1/2 cup of water

1/2 cup of blueberries and apple

1/2 cup of heavy cream

NUTRITION:

Calories: 428

Fat: 42 grams

Carbs: 9 grams

Fiber: 4 grams

Protein: 6 grams

Chocolate Cauliflower Smoothie

INGREDIENTS:

1 cup (240 ml) of unsweetened almond or coconut milk

1 cup (85 grams) of frozen cauliflower florets

1.5 tablespoons (6 grams) of unsweetened cocoa powder

3 tablespoons (30 grams) of hemp seeds

1 tablespoon (10 grams) of cacao nibs

a pinch of sea salt

NUTRITION:

Calories: 316

Fat: 24 grams

Carbs: 15 grams

Fiber: 8 grams

Protein: 16 grams

Pumpkin spice smoothie

INGREDIENTS:

1/2 cup of almond milk or another vegetable milk

1/2 cup of pumpkin purée

2 tablespoons of almond butter

1/4 teaspoon of pumpkin pie spice

1/2 cup of ice

a pinch of sea salt

NUTRITION:

Calories: 464

Fat: 39 grams

Carbs: 19 grams

Fiber: 8 grams

Protein: 12 grams

Key lime pie smoothie

INGREDIENTS:

1 cup (240 ml) of water

1/2 cup (120 ml) of unsweetened almond milk

1/4 cup (28 grams) of raw cashews

1 cup (20 grams) of spinach

2 tablespoons (20 grams) of shredded coconut

2 tablespoons (30 ml) of lime juice

NUTRITION:

Calories: 292

Fat: 24 grams

Carbs: 18 grams

Fiber: 4 grams

Protein: 9 grams

Banana smoothy

INGREDIENTS:

50 g of low-fat ricotta cheese

150 ml of soy milk

20 g of raisins

20 g of almonds

50 g of banana pulp

5 g of wheat bran

20 g of whey protein

1 g guar gum

NUTRITION:

Calories: 296

Fat: 24 grams

Carbs: 23 grams

Fiber: 4 grams

Protein: 11 grams

Creamy cabbage smoothy

INGREDIENTS:

1/2 cup of boiled brown rice

1/2 cup of soy milk

4 leaves of cabbage

4 almonds

the zest of half a lemon grated

a pinch of salt and pepper

NUTRITION:

Calories: 292

Fat: 24 grams

Carbs: 18 grams

Fiber: 4 grams

Protein: 9 grams

Spicy smoothy

INGREDIENTS:

1/2 apple

1/2 mango

1/2 Lemmon

1/2 ripe avocado

2 tender celery stalks

1 kiwi

Almonds to taste

1 pot of Greek yogurt

Oat flakes to taste

a pinch of turmeric

NUTRITION:

Calories: 281

Fat: 23 grams

Carbs: 19 grams

Fiber: 6 grams

Protein: 11 grams

Fresh fennel smoothly

INGREDIENTS:

1 cup of baby spinach

1/2 lime

1/2 fennel

2 tablespoons of fresh goat cheese

2 walnuts

4 almonds

2 tablespoons of oat flakes

a sprig of fennel

a pinch of salt and pepper

NUTRITION:

Calories: 281

Fat: 23 grams

Carbs: 19 grams

Fiber: 6 grams

Protein: 11 grams

Exotic smoothy

INGREDIENTS:

1 carrot

1/2 mango

1/2 papaya

2 tablespoons of Greek yogurt

4 walnuts

1/2 glass of soy milk

the juice of 1/2 orange

wild fennel

a pinch of turmeric

NUTRITION:

Calories: 424

Fat: 38 grams

Carbs: 23 grams

Fiber: 8 grams

Protein: 9 grams

DISHES: PHASE 1 AND 2

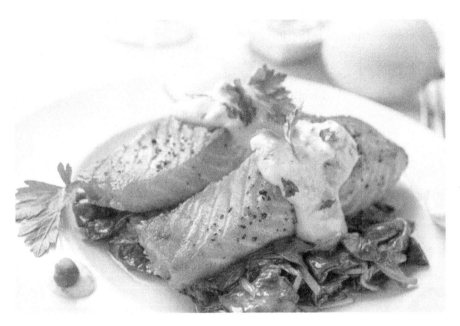

Dear Readers,

I selected the follo

wing creative recipes in order for them to be healthy and full of antioxidant nutrients.

These recipes, combined with smoothies, have a strong slimming power. I recommend you to prepare the recipes with a fair component of carbohydrates for lunch and those with a prevalence of protein in the evening for dinner.

This is because carbohydrates are not easily disposed of in the evening and therefore they get transformed into fat that the body accumulates during the night.

I highly suggest starting lunch and dinner by eating vegetables, especially raw ones because vegetables, being rich in fiber, they not only have a satiating power, but they also help to increase the "good" bacteria that populate our intestines. The positive consequences are:

. a sense of greater satiety 'and satisfaction

. a more efficient intestine

And now......."**Buon Appetito**"!

Avocado, Eggs and Asparagus Tartare

Time required for preparation: 20 minutes

Cooking time: 10 minutes

Serving: 2

Ingredients:

- 250 g of asparagus
- 2 boiled eggs cut into cubes
- 1 lemon
- 4 tablespoons of extra virgin olive oil
- A handful of chopped almonds
- 4 chopped anchovies
- 1 avocado
- A pinch of garlic powder
- Fresh Basil
- Salt and pepper

Preparation:

1. Cook the asparagus for 10 minutes.
2. Emulsify the oil, juice of half lemon, basil and garlic powder.
3. Dice the avocado and drizzle the remaining lemon juice over it so it doesn't darken.
4. Season chopped asparagus, avocado, anchovies, almonds and eggs in a large bowl with the oil emulsion.

5. Prepare the tartare by pouring half of the compost into a ramekin previously placed in the center of the plate.

6. Garnish with basil.

Nutrition:

- Calories in a serving: 440

- 35 g of fat

- Carbohydrates: 5,9 g

- 18 g of protein

Turkey with Tuna Sauce

Time required for preparation: 20 minutes

Cooking time: 10 minutes

Serving: 4

Ingredients:

- 800 g of turkey breast
- 1 onion
- 2 tablespoons of extra virgin olive oil
- 320 g of canned tuna
- 1 cup of water
- 3 anchovy fillets
- 4 hard-boiled eggs, peeled and chopped
- 2 tablespoons of capers brine, soaked in water and drained
- A pinch of salt and pepper

Preparation:

1. sprinkle the turkey with salt and pepper.
2. cut the onion into thin slices. Add into a pot the extra virgin olive oil and heat the onions for 2 minutes.
3. add the turkey and the tuna. Turn the heat up and sear the turkey to cook it on all its sides.
4. add the water and when it comes to a boil, turn down the heat to simmer and cook for 50 minutes, cover to finish cooking
5. remove the turkey from the pot. Take the tuna and the onion separated from the cooking liquid and blend them with anchovy fillets and boiled eggs until very smooth.
6. cut the turkey into thin slices and serve it with the sauce poured over it. Garnish with capers.

Nutrition:

- Calories in a serving: 440

- Fat 29 g

- Carbohydrates: 6,3 g

- Protein 25 g

Marinated Anchovies

Time required for preparation: 15 minutes

Serving: 4

Ingredients:

- 800 g of anchovies fillets already cleaned
- 1 cup of white wine vinegar

- 1 cup of extra-virgin olive oil
- 1/4 cup finely chopped parsley
- 1 garlic clove, sliced paper-thin
- a pinch of sea salt and pepper
- 1 lemon wedges

Preparation:

1. put a layer of the fillets in a baking dish and pour 2 tablespoons of vinegar over it. Layer the rest of the fillets
2. cover the baking dish and marinate it in the fridge for 5 hours
3. rinse, and pat dry the fillets and wash out the baking dish. Replace a layer of anchovies to the dish and sprinkle with 3 tablespoons olive oil, a pinch of salt, pepper, parsley and garlic slices
4. layer in the rest of the anchovies with the same seasoning. cover again and marinate for 1 hour
5. serve the anchovies on each plate with a lemon wedge

Tip:

Serve this dish with avocado slices and whole wheat bread slices

Nutrition:

- Calories in a serving: 428
- Fat 28 g
- Carbohydrates: 1 g
- Protein 33 g

Green Lasagna

Time required for preparation: 20 minutes

Cooking time: 20 minutes

Serving: 4

Ingredients:

- 200 g ready-made pasta for wholemeal lasagna
- 700 ml soy milk
- 40 g of almond flour
- 400 g of zucchini cut into slices
- 70 g of spelt flour
- A pinch of Salt and Pepper
- Nutmeg
- 4 table spoons of Extra virgin olive oil

Preparation:

1. Grill the slices of zucchini and boil the pasta for the lasagna.

2. In another pot combine the flour and soy milk stirring with a whisk to mix well.

3. Add salt, pepper and nutmeg.

4. Bring the béchamel sauce to a boil over low heat, stirring until creamy. Allow to cool.

6. Take a casserole dish and form the layers of lasagna alternating pasta for lasagna, the bechamel sauce and the slices of zucchini. Between each layer add the almond flour.

7.   Finish with a layer of lasagna. Add the oil and the almond flour before placing in the preheated oven at 200 degrees for 20 minutes.

Nutrition:

- Calories in a serving: 350
- 4 g of fat
- Carbohydrates: 59 g
- 19 g of protein

Cabbage Roll with Tuna

Time required for preparation: 10 minutes

Cooking time: 50 minutes

Serving: 4

Ingredients:

- 1 cooked cup of quinoa
- 1 chopped onion
- 1 Finely chopped garlic clove
- 320 g of canned tuna
- one and a half cans of diced tomatoes
- 1/2 cup of fresh minced basil leave
- 8 green whole cabbage leaves
- 2 teaspoons of extra virgin olive oil

Instructions:

1.   Turn on the oven and set it to a temperature of 350 degrees Fahrenheit.

2.   In a non-stick pan, add the extra virgin olive oil, the onion, the quinoa, the garlic and the tuna. Cook for 5 minutes. Add the tomato sauce and basil. Mix well. Continue to cook for another 10 minutes.

3.   Place 2 cabbage leaves on top of the baking sheet. Put a quarter of the filling on top, close the cabbage leaves with kitchen twine. Repeat to make the other three rolls.

4.   Bake in the oven for 40 minutes covered with aluminum foil.

5.   Allow for a 10-minute resting period before serving.

Nutrition:

*   Calories in a serving: 261

*   2 g of fat

*   Carbohydrates: 51 g

*   12 g of protein

Mango, Quinoa, and Chickpeas with Sauce

Time required for preparation: 10 minutes

Servings: 4

Ingredients:

*   2 cups of cooked quinoa

- Drain and rinse 2 cups of chickpeas before using
- 6 leaves of mint
- 1 mango peeled and cut
- 1 avocado peeled and cut
- A pinch of salt
- 2 teaspoons of extra virgin olive oil

Instructions:

1. Combine the chickpeas, mango, avocado, quinoa and fresh mint in a large mixing bowl.
2. Finish by seasoning with salt and oil and serving.

Nutrition:

- 573 calories in a serving
- 23 g of fat
- Carbohydrates: 75 g
- 15 g of protein

Peppers, Onion with Tuna

Time required for preparation: 10 minutes

Cooking preparation: 10 minutes

Serving: 2

Ingredients:

- 2 tablespoons of coconut oil
- 1/2 teaspoon of turmeric
- 2 onions, peeled and finely chopped
- 2 green chilies, finely diced
- 2 tuna fillets
- 2 tablespoons of extra virgin olive oil
- 3 tablespoons of tomato paste
- A pinch of salt
- Washed and sliced 1 red bell pepper

Instructions:

1. Heat the coconut oil in a nonstick skillet. Add turmeric, onion, green chilies and red bell pepper. Cook for 5 minutes.
2. Grill the tuna.
3. Serve the tuna with the vegetables and dress with extra virgin olive oil.

Nutrition:

- Calories in a serving: 520
- Carbohydrates: 81 g
- 8 g fat
- 6 g of dietary fiber
- 4 g of protein

Pizza with Mixed Vegetables

Time required for preparation: 10 minutes

Cooking preparation: 30 minutes

Servings: 4

Ingredients:

For the pizza sauce, use the following ingredients:

- 1 can of diced tomatoes
- 1 tablespoon of extra-virgin olive oil
- ½ a cup of fresh basil leaves, rinsed thoroughly
- 1/2 a garlic peeled and chopped clove
- 1/4 teaspoon of dried sage
- 1 teaspoon of salt

For the pizza, use the following ingredients:

- 4 whole wheat pizza bases
- Shredded mozzarella
- Rinse and thinly slice 1 cup of mixed vegetables of your choice (tomatoes; eggplant; onion; green pepper; mushroom)
- 1/3 cup of finely chopped pitted olives
- 1 tablespoon of extra-virgin olive oil
- 5 basil leaves, washed and split into tiny pieces

Instructions:

1. To prepare the sauce, follow these steps:
2. In a blender, blend on low speed until the basil and garlic are very tiny bits, then add the olive oil and blend until smooth.

3. Put diced tomatoes and salt and cook in a saucepan for about 20 minutes, or until the sauce has reduced somewhat.

To prepare the pizza, follow these steps:

1. Set the oven to 500 degrees Fahrenheit. Prepare a baking sheet by lining it with parchment paper and setting it aside.
2. Spread the pizza sauce over the pizza bases in a uniform layer. Place the mozzarella on top and sprinkle the cut vegetables and olives, the basil and garlic emulsion and dried sage.
3. Bake for about 8 minutes.
4. Drizzle the pizzas with olive oil and sprinkle the basil leaves on top of them to finish. For about three weeks, you can store leftovers in the freezer in an airtight container.

Nutrition:

*   Calories in a serving: 400

*   10 g of total fat

*   Carbohydrates: 64 g

*   5 g of dietary fiber

*   10 g of protein

Chickpeas Chili

Time for preparation: 15 minutes

Cooking time: 30 minutes

Serving: 2

Ingredients:

- 1 tablespoon of coconut oil
- 1 medium-sized onion, peeled and chopped
- 6 mushrooms, cleaned and cut into slices
- 2 tablespoons of freshly ground coriander
- ½ tablespoon of paprika
- ½ teaspoon of chilli powder
- 1 cap of diced tomatoes
- 1 cap of rinsed chickpeas
- 1 cap of rinsed kidney beans
- 2 tablespoons of tomato purée
- 7 oz. of uncooked brown rice
- 4 fresh cilantro sprigs, to be used for garnishing (optional)

Instructions:

1.   Place the coconut oil over medium heat in a large skillet. Add the onion and cook for two minutes then add the mushrooms and cook for another 4 minutes. Combine the paprika and chilli powder until well combined.

2.   Stir in the canned tomatoes and their juices, chickpeas, kidney beans and tomato purée until everything is well-combined. All ingredients should be stirred together and brought to a simmer. Cook for 25 minutes at medium heat.

3.   While the chilli is cooking, prepare the rice according to the directions on the box. Drain after rinsing.

4.   Arrange the chilli on top of the rice, topped with cilantro and serve immediately.

Nutrition:

- Calories in a serving: 580

- 5 g of total fat
- Carbohydrates: 102 g
- 18 g of dietary fibre
- 19 g of protein

Lentils with Sweet Potatoes

Time required for preparation: 10 minutes

Cooking preparation: 30 minutes

Servings: 4

Ingredients:

- 2 tablespoons of coconut oil
- 1 onion, peeled
- 2 carrots peeled and chopped
- 2 celery stalks, washed and chopped
- 1 sweet potato, washed and chopped
- 1 cup cooked lentils
- 5 cups vegetable stock
- A pinch of salt

Instructions:

1. Heat the coconut oil over medium heat. Add the onion and cook for 3 minutes.
2. Add the carrots, celery and sweet potato and continue cooking for another 2 minutes.

3. Pour in the lentils and the vegetable stock. Stir constantly until the lentils are tender, about 25 minutes.
4. Add salt before serving.

Nutrition:

- Calories in a serving: 330

- Carbs: 49 g

- Fat: 10 g

- 20 g of fiber

- 17 g of protein

Pasta with Anchovies and Tomatoes

Time required for preparation: 10 minutes

Cooking time: 35 minutes

Servings: 4

Ingredients:

- Extra-virgin olive oil (around 3 tablespoons)
- 2 garlic cloves, peeled and smashed
- 1 diced onion
- ½ cups of anchovies
- 1 eggplant (rinsed and chopped)
- 2 diced zucchinis
- 4 tomatoes, washed and chopped
- 1 cup of sun-dried tomatoes
- 2 tbsp of dried basil
- 1 tbsp of wine vinegar

- A pinch of salt
- 7 ounces of spelt pasta

Instructions:

1. Over medium heat, shimmer the olive oil in a large skillet. Sauté the garlic, onion, anchovies and eggplant for 8 minutes, or until the eggplant is soft.
2. Add the zucchini, tomatoes, sun-dried tomatoes, salt and basil Cook for 8 minutes.
3. Place the pasta in a separate pot with boiling water cover it and simmer for approximately 10 minutes, or until the pasta is tender but not falling apart.
4. Serve the pasta immediately with the sauce.

Nutrition:

- Calories: 460 per serving
- 12 g of total fat
- Carbohydrates: 75 g
- 17 g of protein

Crispy Green Tomatoes

Time required for preparation: 10 minutes

Cooking time: 15 minutes

Servings: 2

Ingredients:

- 1/4 cup of coconut flour

- Pinch of salt
- 4 sliced green tomatoes
- 1 cup of apple sauce
- 1/2 cup of almond flour
- 1/2 cup of extra-virgin olive oil

Instructions:

1. To begin, combine the coconut flour and salt in a large mixing basin. Toss the tomatoes together. Toss until everything is thoroughly covered.
2. Pour the apple sauce into a separate mixing dish. Toss in the almond flour. Combine until everything is well-combined.
3. Bring the oil to a boil. Dip the tomatoes into the apple sauce mixture. Repeat with the remaining tomatoes. Using batches, fry the tomatoes for about 3 minutes each until golden brown. Serve.

Nutrition:

- Calories in a serving: 113
- Fat: 4.2 g
- Carbohydrates: 22.5 g
- Fiber: 6.3 g
- Protein: 9.2 g

Stir Fry with Zucchini and Broccoli

Time required for preparation: 10 minutes

Cooking time: 10 minutes

Serving: 4

Ingredients:

- 2 tablespoons of coconut oil
- 1 piece of fresh ginger, peeled and finely chopped
- 2 garlic cloves, peeled and minced
- 2 chopped onions
- 1 broccoli head, washed and split into florets
- 1-cup of steamed zucchini, washed and sliced into long
- 1 cup of tuna
- ½ cup of anchovies
- 1 tablespoon of finely chopped fresh basil leaves

Instructions:

1. Heat the coconut oil in a wok or a big pan over medium heat. Add the ginger and garlic. Cook for 3 minutes.
2. Add the onions, tuna, anchovies and broccoli to the pan and simmer for 3 minutes, or until the onion begins to soften a little.
3. Combine the zucchini and basil. Toss everything together and cook for 4 minutes until the veggies are soft.
4. Turn off the heat, transfer to a serving platter and add fresh basil before serving.

Nutrition:

- Calories in a serving: 180

- 14 g of total fat
- Carbohydrates: 13 g
- 3 g of dietary fiber
- 3 g of protein

Kamut Noodles with Walnuts Pesto

Time required for preparation: 5 minutes

Cooking time: 10 minutes

Servings: 2

Ingredients:

- Extra-virgin olive oil (around 3 tablespoons)
- 1 bunch of freshly picked basil leaves
- 1/2 cup of walnuts
- 6 cups of well washed cooked kamut noodles (cooked according to package directions)
- 1 bunch of fresh parsley
- 1 bunch of fresh cilantro
- A pinch of salt

Instructions:

- Combine the olive oil, basil, walnuts, parsley, and cilantro in a blender until well combined. Blend until the mixture is smooth.
- Combine the cooked noodles and the sauce in a large mixing basin. Toss to combine flavours.

Nutrition:

- Calories in a serving: 355

- Total fat: 21

- Carbohydrates: 36 g

- Dietary fiber: 1 g

- Protein: 9 g

Quinoa, Eggs and Bears

Time required for preparation: 10 minutes

Time required for cooking: 20 minutes

Servings: 4

Ingredients:

- 1 cup of quinoa, well washed

- 1 can of rinsed black beans

- 1 teaspoon of cumin seeds

- 2 tablespoons of extra virgin olive oil

- 2 minced garlic cloves

- 2 eggs boiled cut into pieces

- 1 lime (squeezed)

- Avocado thinly sliced

- Fresh cilantro (about one handful)

Instructions:

1.   Pour the quinoa in boiling water and mix. Cook it for about 8 minutes.

2.   While that's happening, in a small skillet combine olive oil, the black beans, garlic and cumin.

3.   Simmer for 10 minutes.

4.   Combine the quinoa, eggs and warmed beans in a large mixing basin until well combined. Place the avocado, lime juice and cilantro over the top and serve immediately.

Nutrition:

- 420 calories per serving

- 9 g of total fat

- Carbohydrates: 70 g

- 18 g of dietary fibre

- 10 g of protein

Salmon with Roasted Vegetables

Time required for preparation: 10 minutes

Cooking time: 30 minutes

Servings: 2

Ingredients:

- 2 cups of olive oil,

- 2 big heads of garlic

- 2 big eggplants
- 2 large shallots peeled, then quartered
- 2 slices of salmon
- 2 carrots, peeled and cut into cubes
- 1 giant parsnip, peeled and cut into cubes
- 1 small green bell pepper
- 1 broccoli
- 1 big sprig of thyme, with plucked leaves
- A pinch of salt

Ingredients for garnishing:

- ½ lemon divided into wedges and ½ squeezed
- 1 / 8 cup fennel bulb, finely chopped

Instructions:

1.   Preheat the oven until the temperature reaches 425 degrees Fahrenheit.

2.   Prepare a deep roasting pan by lining it with aluminum foil and gently greasing it with oil. Toss in all the vegetables, herbs and salt to taste.

3.   Add the remaining oil and lemon juice until well combined. Toss everything together well.

4.   To cover the roasting pan, place a piece of aluminum foil. Place this on the center oven rack and bake for 30 minutes. Remove the aluminum foil from the pan. After cooling for a few minutes, divide evenly among plates.

5.   Finish with a finely chopped fennel bulb and a lemon slice to garnish the dish. Grill the salmon slices and serve with the vegetables. Garnish with lemon juice.

Nutrition:

- Calories in a serving: 164

- Fat: 4.2 g

- Carbohydrates: 22.5 g

- 6.3 g of dietary fiber

- 9.2 grams of protein

Emmer with Lemon Flower

Time required for preparation: 10 minutes

Cooking time: 15 minutes

Servings: 2

Ingredients:

- 1 cup of emmer

- 4 cleaned chopped tomatoes

- Extra-virgin olive oil (around 2 tablespoons)

- 1/4 cup of chopped dried apricot

- 1 teaspoon grated lemon zest

- 1 tbsp lemon juice

- ½ cup of walnuts

- 1/2 cup of finely chopped fresh parsley
- A pinch of salt

Instructions:

1.   Place the emmer in a pot full of water. Boil for 15 minutes and drain.

2.   Combine the olive oil, apricots, lemon zest, lemon juice, walnuts, parsley and and tomatoes in a large mixing bowl. Adjust seasonings if needed, and serve.

Nutrition:

- Calories in a serving: 270
- Fat: 8 g
- Carbohydrates: 42 g
- 5 g of dietary fiber
- 6 g of protein

Swordfish with Onions

Time required for preparation: 10 minutes

Cooking time: 11 minutes

Servings: 4

Ingredients:

- 4 big halved onions
- 2 garlic crushed cloves

- 1/2 a tablespoon of balsamic vinegar

- 4 slices of swordfish

- 1/2 teaspoon of Dijon mustard

- 2 tablespoons of extra virgin olive oil

Instructions:

1.   In a large skillet, combine the oil, onions and garlic. Fry for 1 minute or until the vegetables are tender.

2.   Combine the stock, vinegar and the Dijon mustard.

3.   Make sure the heat is turned down. Simmer the mixture under a cover for 10 minutes.

4.   Continue stirring untill the liquid reduces and the onions have become brown.

5.   Grill the swordfish slices, add the onion sauce and serve.

Nutrition:

- 450 calories per serving

- Fat: 6.4.2 g

- Carbohydrates: 29.5 g

- 16.3 g of dietary fiber

- 19.4 g of protein

Salmon Fillets with Aplle and Onions

Time required for preparation: 10 minutes

Cooking time: 10 minutes

Servings: 2

Ingredients:

- 2 cups of unsweetened apple cider
- 1 big onion, peeled and halved
- 2 fillets of salmon
- 2 apples, peeled and cut into wedges
- A pinch of sea salt

Instructions:

1. In a medium-sized pot, combine the apple cider, onion, apples and salt. Cook until the onion is soft and the liquid has dried.

2. Grill the salmon fillets.

3. Put the onion and apples sauce on the fish and serve.

Nutrition:

- Calories in a serving: 344
- Total fat: 6,5.12 g
- Carbohydrates: 22.5 g
- 6.3 g of dietary fiber
- 9.2 g of protein

Zucchini Noodles with Mushrooms

Time required for preparation: 10 minutes

Cooking time: 4 minutes

Servings: 2

Ingredients:

- 1 zucchini, shredded and made into spaghetti-like strands

- 2 garlic cloves, peeled and minced

- 2 finely sliced white onions

- 2 kilos of mushrooms, cut into thick slicers

- A pinch of sea salt

- 2 tablespoons of coconut oil

- 1 tablespoon of finely chopped fresh chives (for garnish)

Instructions:

1. Melt 2 tablespoons of coconut oil over medium heat in a saucepan. Add the onion, garlic and cook for three minutes, until the onion is soft.

2. Bring the water to a boil. Reduce the heat gradually and allow the zucchini to simmer for 1 minute, drain and add the onion and mushroom sauce.

3 To serve, divide the zucchini noodles into equal portions and arrange them in individual dishes. Top the dish with chives.

Nutrition:

- 256 calories in a serving

- Carbohydrates: 22.5 g

- 6.3 g of dietary fiber

- 4.2 g of protein

Turkey Fillet with Pineapple

Time required for preparation: 12 minutes

Cooking time: 10 minutes

Servings: 2

Ingredients:

- 1 package tempeh (10 ounces, sliced)
- 1/4 pineapple, cut into rings
- Orange juice (about 2 tablespoons, freshly squeezed)
- Freshly squeezed lemon juice (about 1 tablespoon)
- 2 turkey fillet
- 1 tablespoon of extra virgin olive oil

Instructions:

1. Combine the olive and coconut oil, orange and lemon juice in a large mixing bowl. Put the tempeh to marinate in the bowl for e few minutes.

2. Heat a grill pan over medium-high heat. Take the marinated tempeh out of the bowl with a pair of tongs and place it on the grill pan after it has reached a high temperature.

3. Grill for 3 minutes.

4. Slice the pineapple, grill it for a few minutes and place it on a serving plate.

5.   Grill the turkey fillets

6.   Place the grilled turkey, tempeh and pineapple on a serving tray and serve.

Nutrition:

- 329 calories per serving

- Fats: 4.2 g

- Carbohydrates: 22.5 g

- 6.3 g of dietary fiber

- 12.5 g of protein

Eggs and Courgettes with Apple Cider Sauce

Time required for preparation: 10 minutes

Cooking time: 10 minutes

Servings: 2

Ingredients:

- 2 cups of courgettes (cut in half)

- 2 tbsps of apple cider vinegar

- 4 tbsps of extra virgin olive oil

- 4 boiled eggs cut into pieces

- 2 Onions, thinly cut

- A piece of grated ginger root (fresh or dried)

Instructions:

1.   To begin grill the courgette slices

2.   While that is going on, in a saucepan, add the apple cider vinegar, oil, onions and ginger root. Cook for 5 minutes.

3.   Put the courgettes in a serving dish with the eggs Add the onion source over the top. Serve

Nutrition :

•   Calories: 378 per serving

•   9.2 g of total fat

•   Carbohydrates: 22.5 g

•   Fiber: 6.3

•   11,4 g of protein

Lamb Ribs with Mixed Mushrooms

Time required for preparation: 5 minutes

Cooking time: 5 minutes

Servings: 2

Ingredients:

•   2 cups of mixed mushrooms

•   2 shallots

•   1 garlic clove

•   2 sprigs of fresh thyme

- 4 lamb ribs
- 2 tablespoons of extra-virgin olive oil
- 2 bay leaves

Instructions:

1. Finely chop the peeled garlic.

2. Chop the mixed mushrooms into small pieces and wash them well.

3. In a large skillet, combine the oil, the shallots, the garlic and the bay leaves. Fry for 1 minute and add the mushrooms, salt and pepper. Cook it for 15 minutes.

4. Grill the lamb ribs.

5. Season with fresh thyme and serve all together.

Nutrition:

- Calories in a serving: 324
- Total fat: 4.6
- Carbohydrates: 22.5 g
- 6.3 g of fiber
- 14.6 g of protein

Proteic Wrap With Shrimps, Avocado and Corn

Time required for preparation: 10 minutes

Cooking time: 2 minutes

Servings: 2

Ingredients:

- 2 wraps
- 100 g of cleaned shrimps
- 30 g of avocado
- 1 tablespoon of corn
- 50 g rocket leaves
- salt, pepper, lime, paprika or herbs to taste

Instruction:

1. Blanch the shrimp (if you want to, you can quickly stir-fry them in a pan with oil and paprika, to give an extra touch of flavor).
2. Mash the avocado (if you want to, you can season it with salt, pepper and lime) and drain and rinse the corn.
3. Heat the wrap on a non-stick pan for 1 minute per side.
4. Put the wraps on a plate and place the filling in the center of it.
5. Close the wraps by rolling them up.

Nutrition:

- Calories in a serving: 265
- Total fat: 6.4 g
- Carbohydrates: 20 g

- 6.3 g of fiber

- 24.6 g of protein

Spicy Soap with Sweet Potatoes

Time required for preparation: 10 minutes

Cooking time: 27 minutes

Servings: 2

Ingredients:

- A teaspoon of grated fresh ginger

- 1 teaspoon of turmeric

- 2 sweet potatoes

- 1 chopped onion

- 4 carrots, peeled and cut into chunks

- 2 tablespoons of extra virgin olive oil

- 2 zucchini

- 1 liter of vegetarian broth

- 1 tablespoon of pumpkin seeds

Instructions:

1.   Cook the onion with the olive oil for 2 minutes.

2.   Add the other all ingredients and bring to a boil for 25 minutes.

3.   Mix them with an immersion blender until you get a smooth and creamy mixture.

4.   If desired, sprinkle some pumpkin seeds on top of the dish as a garnish.

Nutrition:

- Calories in 210 per serving
- 8.2 g of fat
- Carbohydrates: 12.5 g
- Fiber: 5.3 g
- Protein: 8.6 g

Mozzarella Cheese with Salad De Kale

Time required for preparation: 10 minutes

Servings: 2

Ingredients:

- 1 avocado cut into slices
- 1 head of kale, washed, dried and thinly sliced
- 2 fresh mozzarella cheese cut into pieces
- 4 fresh basil leaves
- 2 tablespoons of extra-virgin olive oil
- A few pumpkin seeds
- A pinch of salt and pepper

Instructions:

1. Put in a salad bowl the avocado, the mozzarella cheese and the kale.

2 Add all the dressing ingredients.

3. Season with the pumpkin seeds and the basil.

4. Serve.

Nutrition:

- Calories in a serving: 356

- Fat: 8.2 g

- Carbohydrates: 13.5 g

- Fiber: 3.3 g

- Protein: 9.2 g

Italian Minestrone Soap

Time required for preparation: 15 minutes

Cooking time: 27 minutes

Servings: 2

The "Hearty Minestrone" is packed with alkaline nutrients and it is also unbelievably delicious. By preparing it you simply perform an excellent service for your body. This vegetable minestrone is a good source of minerals and fiber; it also contains various vitamins and phytonutrients, which act as antioxidants.

The mix of carrots, zucchini, and sweet potatoes contained in this dish leaves no question to the fact that it is tasty, nutritious, and healthful.

Ingredients:

- 4 fresh basil leaves
- 1 carrot
- 2 zucchini
- 2 sweet potatoes cut into pieces
- 1 chopped red onion
- 2 tablespoons of extra virgin olive
- 1 liter of vegetable broth
- 1 cup of tomato juice
- 1/2 cup of cooked beans
- A pinch of Black pepper and Himalayan salt

Instructions:

1. For 2 minutes, heat the oil in a large pan and fry the onion, carrot and zucchini.

2. Stir in the tomato juice, stock, and beans until well combined.

3. Bring the mixture to a boil, add the mashed sweet potatoes and decrease the heat to a low level; cook for 25 minutes. Add the salt and the pepper.

4. Add the fresh basil and serve.

Nutrition:

Calories in a serving: 110

Fat: 6.4 g

Carbohydrates: 11.3 g

Fiber: 3.5 g

Protein: 5.6 g

Spicy Zucchini and Carrots Noodles

Time required for preparation: 15 minutes

Cooking time: 1 minutes

Servings: 2

Ingredients:

- 2 medium-sized zucchinis

- 2 carrots

- 1 tablespoon of coconut oil

- 1 tablespoon of fresh chopped coriander freshly

- A piece of grated ginger root

- 2 teaspoons of lemon or lime juice

- 1/4 cup of almond butter

Instructions:

1. Begin with the courgette and carrot noodles, which should be sliced thinly using a mandolin or vegetable peeler.

2. For the sauce, combine the ginger, the coconut oil, the garlic, the lime/lemon juice, the almond butter in a blender.

3. Pour in a bit of water and blend until a thick sauce is created.

4. Boil the courgette and the carrot noodles for 1 minute.

5. Finally, obtain a large mixing basin and combine the zucchini and carrots noodles with the sauce.

6. Garnish with a coriander.

Nutrition:

Calories in a serving: 229

Fat: 6.2 g

Carbohydrates: 13.7 g

Fiber: 6.2 g

Protein: 6.4 g

Quinoa, Spinach whit Lime

Time required for preparation: 10 minutes.

Cooking time: 17 minutes.

Servings: 4

Ingredients:

- 2 cups of quinoa

- 2 cups of water

- 1 sweet potato thinly sliced

- 1 teaspoon of turmeric

- 1 tbsp. of ground cumin seeds

- 1/2 teaspoon of freshly grated ginger

- 1 cup of finely chopped onion

- 2 tablespoons of extra-virgin olive oil

- A pinch of salt and pepper

Instructions:

1. Put the onion and the olive oil in to the pan and cook for 2 minutes.

2. Stir in the ginger, sweet potatoes, turmeric, quinoa and the 2 cups of water.

3. Cook for 15 minutes.

4. Put on plates, serve, and garnish with cumin seeds.

Nutrition:

Calories in a serving: 268

Fat: 9.9 g

Carbohydrates: 38.8 g

Protein content: 7.6 g

Soup with Mixed Mushrooms

Time required for preparation: 15 minutes

Cooking time: 50 minutes

Serving: 2

Ingredients:

- 3 cups of Mushrooms
- 1 cup of Beans
- 1 cup of kale, finely chopped
- 2 tomatoes, peeled and sliced
- Chopped (about 1/2 cup) red onions
- A pinch of Himalayan Pink Salt
- 4 fresh basil leaves
- A pinch of oregano
- 2 tablespoons of extra virgin olive oil

Instructions:

1. Put all the ingredients in a saucepan and cook over low heat for 50 minutes.
2. Let it cool and mix everything with an immersion blender.
3. Serve the mushroom soup in bowls and enjoy!

Tip:

To accompany the Mushroom Soup, you can serve it with Tortillas or Herb Bread.

Nutrition:

Calories in a serving: 240

Fat: 2.4 g

Carbohydrates: 11.3 g

Fiber: 3.5 g

Protein: 5.3 g

Soup with Tomatoes, Beans and Oregano Leaves

Time required for preparation: 10 minutes

Cooking time: 55 minutes

Serving: 2

Ingredients:

- 3 cups of Beans
- 4 tomatoes, finely chopped
- Green Bell Pepper (1/2 cup)
- 1 chopped onion
- A pinch of salt and pepper
- 4 fresh basil leaves
- A pinch of of oregano leaves
- 2 tablespoons of extra virgin olive oil

Instructions:

1. Place the olive oil, the tomatoes, the onion, the bell peppers in a large pot. Sauté vegetables for 4–5 minutes on medium heat, stirring occasionally.

2. Add the beans, 1 cup of water, salt and pepper.

3. Cook for approximately 50 minutes on a low heat setting.

4. Dish up your Spicy Tomato Bean Soup and garnish with oregano leaves.

Nutrition:

Calories in a serving: 210

Fat: 6.4 g

Carbohydrates: 15.3 g

Fiber: 4.6 g

Protein: 8.9 g

Soup with Asparagus

Time required for preparation: 10 minutes

Cooking time: 15 minutes

Servings: 2

Ingredients:

- 2 lb. fresh asparagus trimmed off woody stems
- 1 teaspoon of dried thyme
- ½ teaspoon of dried oregano
- 1 cauliflower head, florets removed from the head
- 1 tablespoon of minced garlic
- 1 leek, thinly sliced
- 1 tablespoon of coconut oil

- A pinch of salt and pepper

Instructions:

1. Boil the asparagus, leek and cauliflower in a large pot filled with water.

2. Heat the coconut oil in a large pot. Add the cooked vegetables, herbs and lime juice. Cook for 10 minutes, mixing frequently.

3. Turn off the heat and blend everything with an immersion blender.

4. Allow to cool and serve on plates.

Nutrition:

Calories in a serving: 110

Fat: 6.4 g

Carbohydrates: 11.3 g

Fiber: 3.5 g

Protein: 5.6 g

Salad with Watercress and Mixed Seeds

Preparation time: 10 minutes

Servings: 2

Ingredients:

- 2 cucumbers cut into slices

- ½ cup of green olives

- 2 cups of watercress, torn into pieces
- 1 lime zest and 2 tablespoons lime juice
- 4 cutlery nuts into small pieces
- 4 fresh basil leaves
- 1/2 teaspoon of turmeric powder
- 2 tbsp. of sunflower seeds, chia seeds and pumpkin seeds
- 2 tablespoons of extra-virgin olive oil
- A pinch of Himalayan Pink Salt

Instructions:

1. Combine the olive oil and key lime juice in a large salad bowl. Mix them thoroughly to ensure that they are well-combined.
2. Add the thinly sliced vegetables, olives, walnuts, turmeric, lime zest, salt and herbs.
3. Dish up and enjoy your quick and easy Fresh Salad!

Nutrition:

Calories in a serving: 92

Fat: 2.4 g

Carbohydrates: 11.3 g

Fiber: 6.5 g

Protein: 4.6 g

Squash Salad

Preparation time: 10 minutes

Servings: 2

Ingredients:

- 4 zucchini cut into thin slices
- 1/2 cup of Brazil Nuts that have been soaked (overnight or at least 4 hours)
- 1/4 cup of coconut milk
- A quarter teaspoon of finely chopped dates
- A pinch of Himalayan Pink Salt and pepper
- 2 teaspoons of lime juice

Instructions:

1. Put the thinly sliced zucchini in a salad bowl.
2. In a blender, combine the dates, coconut milk and Brazil nuts. Blend until smooth.
3. Season the vegetables with the blended emulsion, lime juice, salt and pepper
4. Serve immediately.

Nutrition:

Calories in a serving: 110

Fat: 2.6 g

Carbohydrates: 11.5 g

Fiber: 3.5 g

Protein: 6.5 g

Mango Salad and Red Onion

Preparation time: 10 minutes

Size of each serving: 2

Ingredients:

- 6 plum tomatoes
- 1/2 cup of mango chunks (diced)
- 1 tomatillo (tomatillos are a type of tomato).
- red onions (about half a cup diced)
- 1/4 cup of chopped Green Bell Peppers
- Cilantro leaves (about 1/2 cup)
- A pinch of Himalayan Pink Salt
- A pinch of onion powder
- 2 teaspoons of lime juice
- 2 tablespoons of extra virgin olive oil

Instructions:

1. Cut all the vegetables thin and put them in a salad bowl.
2. Add the mango, lime juice and seasonings
3. Enjoy your Quick Mango Salad!

Nutrition:

Calories in a serving: 110

Fat: 1.4 g

Carbohydrates: 15.3 g

Fiber: 2.5 g

Protein: 6.4 g

Salad de Chickpeas with Mayonnaise

Time required for preparation: 15 minutes plus 30 minutes in the refrigerator

Serving: 4

Ingredients:

- 2 cups of chickpeas that have been cooked
- Mayonnaise (about ½ cup)
- Red onions, roughly chopped (about 1/4 cup)
- 1/2 cup of chopped Green Bell Peppers
- 1 teaspoon of Dill
- A pinch of onion powder
- A pinch of Himalayan Pink Salt

Instructions:

1. In a large bowl, combine chickpeas and mayonnaise. Mix.

2. Blend all remaining ingredients and pour them into the salad bowl with the chickpeas. Mix up.

3. Refrigerate it for 30 minutes before serving.

4. Toss the Chickpea Salad together and serve.

Nutrition:

Calories in a serving: 115

Fat: 5.4 g

Carbohydrates: 11.3 g

Fiber: 4.5 g

Protein: 6.4 g

Salad with Sweet Potatoes and Brazil Nuts

Time required for preparation: 10 minutes plus 30 minutes in the refrigerator

Cooking time: 15 minutes

Ingredients:

- 2 sweet potatoes

- 2 zucchini

- 1 carrot

- 1 cup of Brazil Nuts that have been soaked (overnight or at least 4 hours)

- 1/4 cup of sliced Green Bell Peppers

- 1 tablespoon of lime juice

- 4 tablespoons of extra virgin olive oil

- A pinch of Salt and pepper

- A pinch of Ginger Powder

Instructions:

1. 1 In a blender, combine the Brazil Nuts, olive Oil, Lime Juice, spices, ginger powder, salt, pepper and 1/2 cup of water until smooth.

2. Boil carrot, sweet potatoes, and zucchini: let them cool and cut them into slices.

3. Combine everything in a salad bowl, add the green bell peppers and mix.

4. Allow 30 minutes of cooling time in the refrigerator before serving.

5. Plate your "Potato" Salad and enjoy it immediately!

Nutrition:

Calories in a serving: 274

Fat: 5.4 g

Carbohydrates: 19.3 g

Fiber: 5.6 g

Protein: 5.4 g

Beans and Spicy Tomato Sauce

Time required for preparation: 10 minutes

Cooking time: 42 minutes

Serving: 4

Ingredients:

- 6 chopped tomatoes
- 3 cups of Beans
- 1/2 cup of sliced Green Bell Peppers
- 1 diced Onion
- A pinch of Salt
- A piece of freshly grated ginger
- A pinch of turmeric powder
- 2 tablespoons of extra virgin olive oil

To garnish: 4 fresh basil leaves

Instructions:

1. Put the onion, the green bell peppers and oil in a large pot and cook for 2 minutes
2. Add all the other ingredients and continue cooking for another 40 minutes
3. Place on plates and add basil leaves.
4. Serve.

Nutrition:

Calories in a serving: 110

Fat: 6.4 g

Carbohydrates: 11.3 g

Fiber: 3.5 g

Protein: 4.6 g

Fresh Cucumber with Creamy Avocado

Preparation time: 10 minutes plus 20 minutes in the refrigerator

Serving: 2

Ingredients:

- 2 cucumbers cut into thin slices
- 1 ripe avocado cut into pieces
- 1 handful of Basil,
- A pinch of Salt
- 2 tablespoons of extra virgin olive oil
- 1 tablespoons of balsamic vinegar

Instructions:

1. Put the cucumbers in a plate.
2. Place the avocado, oil, salt, basil and vinegar in a blender. Add the salt and purée until smooth.
3. Put the puree to cool in the refrigerator for around 20 minutes.
4. Garnish the cucumbers with avocado cream and serve.

Nutrition:

Calories in a serving: 135

Fat: 2.4 g

Carbohydrates: 11.3 g

Fiber: 3.5 g

Protein: 4.6 g

SNACKS: PHASE 1/ 2 /3

Good and healthy snacks are:

- a few slices of fresh coconut
- a handful of dried fruits such as walnuts, almonds, hazelnuts, etc.
- a piece of dark chocolate
- a small cup of berries

Flaxseed Crackers

Serving: 4

Ingredients:

- 200 g millet or spelt flour
- 35 g of extra virgin olive oil
- a pinch of dried chives
- 60 g of flax seeds
- 200 ml of water
- a pinch of salt

Preparation:

1. Put all the ingredients in a large bowl, mix everything with your hands until you get a homogeneous dough.

2. Give the dough the shape of a ball, wrap it in plastic wrap and refrigerate for about two hours.

3.   Heat the oven to 200 degrees.

4.   Roll out the dough on baking paper and give it the shape of a rectangle with a fairly thin thickness.

5.   Place the dough in an oven dish and with a knife cut it into squares the size of crackers.

6.   Bake for about ten minutes.

7.   Remove from the oven and allow the crackers to cool before removing them from each other.

Nutrition:

- Calories in a serving: 195
- 11 g of fat
- Carbohydrates: 20 g
- 11 g of protein

Baked Crispy Chickpeas

Serving: 2

Ingredients:

- 250 g of precooked chickpeas
- 30 g of rice flour
- 30 ml of olive oil
- A pinch of paprika
- A pinch of dried rosemary
- A pinch of salt

Preparation:

1. Transfer the chickpeas to a bowl and add the paprika, rosemary and mix well with a spoon. Add the flour, salt and olive oil and continue to mix well.
2. Transfer the chickpeas to a baking sheet with parchment paper. Bake them in the oven at 180 degrees for about 20 minutes.

They are crispy and super tasty!

Nutrition:

Calories in a serving: 135

Fat: 1.4 g

Carbohydrates: 11.3 g

Fiber: 6.5 g

Protein: 4.6 g

Spicy Chocolate Breadsticks

Serving: 2

Ingredients:

- 8 Breadsticks
- 150 gr of dark chocolate
- A pinch of chili powder

Preparation:

1. Melt the chocolate in the microwave.
2. Combine the tip of a teaspoon of chili powder with the chocolate and stir.
3. Pour the chocolate into a tall glass and let it cool a bit for 3-4 minutes.
4. Dip half of the breadsticks in the melted chocolate and let them dry for a few moments.

Nutrition:

Calories in a serving: 230

Fat: 2.4 g

Carbohydrates: 11.3 g

Fiber: 3.5 g

Protein: 4.6 g

Coffee Snack

Preparation time: 30 minutes

Serving: 4

Ingredients:

- 4 whole wheat spelt toasts or 4 dry spelt cookies
- 1 cup of pumpkin puree made by steaming pumpkin cut into pieces
- 2 tablespoons agave syrup
- 4 tablespoons of Soy Milk
- 2 cups of coffee

- Bitter cocoa

Instructions:

1. Blend the pumpkin with soy milk and agave syrup
2. Place the rusks on the bottom of a mug a -single portion.
3. Pour over the cups of coffee.
4. Cover with the pumpkin cream and level of well.
5. Sprinkle with unsweetened cocoa powder.

Nutrition:

Calories in a serving: 235

Fat: 2.4 g

Carbohydrates: 9.3 g

Fiber: 4.5 g

Protein:5.6 g

DESSERTS WITH LOW GLYCEMIC INDEX: PHASE 2/3

Cocoa Cream

Preparation time: 5 minutes

Serving: 2

Ingredients:

- 100 gr agave syrup
- 40 gr of cocoa powder
- 5 gr of vanilla powder
- 50 gr almond or soy milk
- a pinch of cinnamon

Instructions:

1. mix all ingredients except cinnamon vigorously.
2. Sprinkle cinnamon to taste.

Tips:

You can add more milk and heat it to obtain a delicious hot drink.

You can serve with Fexseed Crackers

Nutrition:

Calories in a serving: 230

Fat: 2.4 g

Carbohydrates: 11.3 g

Fiber: 3.5 g

Protein: 4.6 g

Rice Bread and Chocolate

Preparation time: 30 minutes

Serving: 4

Ingredients:

- 300 grams of dark chocolate min 85 %.
- 150 grams of rice crackers
- 200 grams of soy milk
- 200 grams of dried fruit
- 1 teaspoon of cinnamon powder
- 1 teaspoon of turmeric powder

Instructions:

1. chop the galettes and the dried fruit together.
2. Heat up the chocolate
3. Add the soy milk and the chopped biscuits and dried fruit.
4. mix well and pour everything on a sheet of baking paper.

5. wrap the baking paper into a cylinder and roll up the ends to close it.

6. Chill the roll in the fridge for at least 2 hours.

7. unroll and cut the chocolate salami into slices.

Nutrition:

Calories in a serving: 265

Fat: 2.4 g

Carbohydrates: 9.3 g

Fiber: 3.5 g

Protein: 4.6 g

Chocolate Cream

Preparation time: 15 minutes

Serving: 4

Ingredients:

- 400 grams of cooked black beans
- 1/2 cup of beloved cocoa
- 3 cups of almond milk
- a tablespoon of agave syrup
- one teaspoon of cinnamon powder
- crumbled dried fruit
- garnish with sliced strawberries

Instructions:

1. Place all ingredients in a large bowl and blend with an immersion blender

2. Divide the cream into 4 cups and chill them in the refrigerator for an hour.

3. Garnish with slices of strawberries.

Nutrition:

Calories in a serving: 230

Fat: 2.4 g

Carbohydrates: 8.3 g

Fiber: 3.6 g

Protein: 4.2 g

Yogurt Cake

Preparation time: 15 minutes

Serving: 4

Ingredients:

- 1 jar of vegetable yogurt 125 g

- 1 jar of sunflower oil

- 1/2 a jar of agave syrup

- 1 jar of almond or soy milk

- 1 jar of spelt flour

- 1 jar of rice flour

- 1 tablespoon of unsweetened cocoa

- 1 sachet of baking powder

Ingredients:

1. Empty the yogurt jar into a large bowl.

2. Add all the other ingredients except for the cocoa and mix well until you get a creamy mixture.

3. Divide the dough into two bowls and in one add the bitter cocoa and stir well.

4. Line a cake tin with baking paper and pour the dough of the first bowl in it then pour the other cacao dough in the center of the cake tin.

5. Bake at 180 degrees for 25 minutes.

Nutrition:

Calories in a serving: 195

Fat: 1.9 g

Carbohydrates: 11.3 g

Fiber: 3.5 g

Protein: 4.6 g

Page intentionally left blank

BOOK 2: THE ANTI-INFLAMMATORY DIET

A PHILOSOPHY OF LIFE. CLEAN EATING FOR LONG LIFE HEALTH. SPECIAL RECIPES INCLUDING DELICIOUS CHOCOLATE DESSERTS AND A 14-DAY DETOX MEAL PLAN

INTRODUCTION

Numerous studies claim that the diet that has the most anti-inflammatory power is a plant-based diet.

The plant-based diet has been one of the most searched for on the Google search engine in recent years.

It's a rather disputed diet by "traditional nutritionists" because it doesn't perfectly comply with the World Health Organization's guidelines on the subject of proper nutrition.

It is certain that topics related to diets have long been the subject of attention for a large part of the world's population.

It is also true that despite the growth in economic well-being compared to the past, we are faced with a generation of people who fall ill at a young age. We only think about food intolerances, allergies to pollen, drugs, powder and certain foods; were as we should think more about how much the number of obese or overweight people has increased in the last fifty years, as well as the incidence of autoimmune, cancer and heart diseases.

We are people who have averagely increased our life expectancy but after already 40-50 years of age we begin to take medicine that will accompany us for life.

At a certain point, people start asking themselves questions and probably wonder if by any chance the cause of their illnesses and the burdening of their bodies is not caused by what they eat.

A plant based diet may be the answer to these questions.

An important principle must not be forgotten: the life force of the human body and its capacity for self-healing.

CHARACTERISTICS OF A PLANT-BASED DIET

A PHILOSOPHY OF LIFE

For some time now, one of the food trends that has received the most attention is the vegetable-based diet.

This type of diet represents more of a philosophy of life than a simple diet based on the principle that food is not only "fuel" but above all "care" for the body.

Food and psychophysical well-being are united in a very close, practically inseparable, relationship.

Mind. A well-balanced, clean diet helps fight the negative emotions we are used to living with such as anxiety, panic, and depression.

Proper nutrition helps us regain control of our emotions.

Body. When you regain control of your body you can also regain control of your metabolism and your weight.

This diet's main purpose is to detoxify and restore new energy to body and mind giving us the possibility to improve our present health.

We must not forget that improving the condition of our present health means preserving our future health.

This diet balances macronutrients - carbohydrates, proteins and fats - with micronutrients – vitamins, minerals, and fibers - of exclusively plant origin.

Preservative-rich, refined, industrially processed, and canned foods are not allowed.

This diet is defined as "electric-alkalizing" because it's based on foods "vibrant with life" and "pure from industrial contamination".

Moreover, this kind of diet has a strong anti-inflammatory power achieved through a deep detoxification of the body.

The properties of the alkalizing and anti-inflammatory diet will be explained in two dedicated chapters of this book.

A HEALTHY CHOICE

By now, there's no denying the close relationship between health and nutrition. The best medicine you can take is food.

We can give a great contribution to our health by choosing the right food just as we can also create the best conditions for the development of disease by choosing a wrong diet.

A good part of the scientific literature now agrees on the benefits that a vegetable based diet is able to generate.

The American Dietetic Association affirmed that a correctly balanced plant-based diet is healthy, adequate from a nutritional point of view and brings health benefits both in the prevention and treatment of many diseases.

Any diet, even an omnivorous one, should include a significant proportion of plant-based foods.

Nutritional recommendations for the prevention of chronic degenerative diseases suggest a diet rich in fruits vegetables, legumes whole grains and low in salt, sugar, and alcohol.

These foods rich in polyphenols, vitamins and minerals have the power to turn off inflammation, alkalize our bodies and have powerful and well-organized immune defenses.

Foods of vegetable origin also contain a lot of fiber that:

- properly nourish the intestinal flora

- transform the intestinal flora from putrefactive to fermentative

- purify the organism from toxic metabolites

Later on we will deepen the correlation between plant-based diet, alkaline pH, inflammation and immune system.

HISTORICAL ORIGINS OF VEGANISM

A plaint based diet can be defined as a vegan diet.

Many are led to believe that veganism is a fairly young reality, but in fact veganism started in the distant 1847 in Ramsgate (England), with the founding of the Vegetarian Society, the oldest vegetarian organization in the world. In the early twenties, this association found itself divided into two factions: associates who preferred a vegetarian diet and those who refused the consumption of dairy products and other derivatives of animal origin.

Thus was born the Vegan Society and the term Vegan, which is the result of some of the first three letters with the last two of the word "Vegetarian".

In 1945, the magazine "The Vegan" already had 500 subscribers and vegan thinking spread quickly, managing to spread a new awareness linked not only to food but also to various issues related to the environment, respect for animals and social coexistence.

A real cultural revolution, a change of course in the way of approaching everything that surrounds us, a real philosophy that in a short time also managed to involve the natural medicine field, agriculture and studies on nutrition.

In 1970 this movement also aroused the interest in "official" medicine, so much so as to encourage the start of new research, especially in the USA, which led to demonizing diets based on animal fats and proteins, defining them as harmful to health.

In 2010 a significant percentage of the world population adopted the vegan philosophy and all of this was also facilitated by a greater possibility of accessing food resources that were previously difficult to find.

I don't want to go into the merits of what kind of diet is more or less "ethical". This is not the purpose of this book.

People who choose to be vegan do so not only for moral reasons but also because they are convinced that only a certain type of vegan food could have the effect of not making people sick and even healing their illnesses if they were already sick.

In general, my thought is that a diet must be sustainable over time, be a pleasant habit that originates from a conscious choice. In other words, the way we eat must become part of our way of being and our lifestyle.

Whatever your dietary orientation is, whether or not it excludes foods of animal origin, what is certain is that plaint based diet has proven to be a valid choice also as a detox plan to be followed occasionally during the year: for example, two weeks every three to four months.

At the end of the book you will find a proper 14-day meal plan after the recipes.

A DIET THAT CAN BE DEFINED AS ANTI-INFLAMMATORY

By the most recent evolutionary theories, inflammation appears to be one of the most effective ways in which the body responds to various external and internal stimulus.

Without a good inflammatory response, not even a trivial wound could heal.

Inflammation, as well as stress, must be an emergency response that is as necessary in the short term as it is deleterious if permanently active.

 So when it becomes a permanent and systemic state, inflammation itself becomes the cause of many modern pathologies such as cardiovascular diseases, hypertension, diabetes, dementia, obesity, tumors, autoimmune diseases, etc.

As written in the famous magazine "Science", having identified inflammation as the pathophysiological mechanism that triggers all chronic diseases, is one of the most important insights that medicine has had in the last twenty years.

Most of the population suffers from a latent inflammation that remains in the shade seemingly harmless.

A diet based on a prevalence of foods containing lactose, gluten, omega 6 (such as sunflower oil and in general most foods processed by the food industry) and sugars, triggers the onset of a latent inflammation destined to become chronic.

Obesity itself causes inflammation, generating a vicious phenomenon for which inflammation makes weight loss more difficult. We will talk about overweight in a separate chapter.

Numerous studies worldwide have tried to circumscribe those nutrients that an anti-inflammatory diet cannot ignore. For example, the important study published in 2010 by the Nutrition Journal that studied the antioxidants contained in 3100 foods used worldwide.

In summary, in the drafting of an anti-inflammatory diet what must be considered is that it will not be a single food that will be effective, nor a single supplement but rather it will be the synergy between foods that contain different antioxidant molecules to counteract inflammation.

An example of an anti-inflammatory food plan resulting from the research mentioned above is structured as follows:

- 5 portions of fruit and vegetables with high antioxidant power (berries, red plums, spinach, broccoli etc.);
- 2 servings of hot drinks such as herbal teas;
- 1 squeezed portion of citrus fruit;
- Vegetable oils such as extra virgin olive oil;
- Foods rich in omega 3 like nuts, avocados.

PLANT BASED DIET IS AN ALKALINE DIET

A healthy diet that aims to maintain the acid-base balance of our body: this is what an alkaline diet is.

The pH allows us to keep the acid-base balance of our body under control, expressing it through a precise value.

PH is measured on a scale ranging from 1 to 14 (we are talking about acid PH for values below 7 and basic PH for higher values). To distinguish which foods are acidic from alkaline ones you should measure their pH after digestion. Assuming that the bloodstream PH level is slightly acidic in order to maintain our acid-base balance at an optimal level, it is advisable to give priority to alkaline foods.

On what principles can food be considered acidic based or alkaline based?

To determine foods basic acid level, the ash that remains after the food is digested is analyzed.

It is important to emphasize that there are foods that are classified as acidic based but which in fact, after a series of chemical reactions that activate digestion, are transformed into alkaline based. This is what normally happens in healthy subjects. The best known indicator to measure the PH level of a food is the Potential Renal Acid Load also called PRAL index. This index divides foods into two categories:

- foods with PRAL + have an acidifying effect (such as dairy products, fish, eggs, meat and fish).
- foods with PRAL - are alkalizing (fruits and vegetables).

An alkaline diet, very appreciated in alternative medicine, prefers above all basic foods (also called "alkaline" foods), including various varieties of vegetables and fruit that should be eaten raw if possible to maintain the large quantities of basic minerals they contain (calcium, magnesium and potassium).

Scientific studies have shown how much alkaline foods are beneficial both on our metabolism and on the health of our intestine due to their power to rebalance the intestinal microbiota.

Wanting to choose to drastically lower the acidity level of our body, it is possible to practice alkaline fasting which is an extreme form of this diet. In this case, only alkaline foods are taken, while for drinks you should only drink water and herbal infusions. However, some nutritionists advise against following this practice in the long term, as it could generate important nutritional deficiencies.

How important is the acid-base balance in our body?

Now we begin to approach the crucial point of understanding why so many choose to follow an alkaline diet. The reason is simple: this diet affects our acid-base balance. Those who follow a diet of this type will therefore avoid reaching too high levels of acidity in the body.

But what exactly is meant by acid-base balance?

In a nutshell, it's the relationship between acidity and alkalinity within the body.

As a matter of fact, our body is equipped with a mechanism called "buffer system", which tries to regulate the correct acid-base balance of the body, preventing dangerous imbalances and variations in acidity and alkalinity from being generated.

However, if we follow a diet made mainly of acidic foods, the buffer system may lose efficiency and a situation of hyperacidity occurs.

In this case, various ailments and diseases such as fatigue, digestive problems, migraines, muscle or joint pains can occur.

So if it is true that our buffer system works autonomously, it is also true that it must not be put under too much strain and, at least occasionally, it also needs to be regenerated.

A DIET THAT STRENGTHENS THE IMMUNE SYSTEM

The immune system is the body's first line of defense, the rapid response mechanism against the attack of pathogens. Having weak immune defenses, therefore, means being more exposed to diseases and infections.

To influence this defense mechanism is mainly the intestine: think that 80% of the cells responsible for the functioning of the immune system are found in the intestine.

Inside, the intestine is populated by entire colonies of microorganisms that make up the microbiota. A balanced microbiota guarantees us to stay away from that dangerous and latent general inflammatory state that exposes us to a greater risk of getting sick.

Various studies have shown how an alkaline and anti-inflammatory diet, such as a paint based diet, affects the strength and efficiency of our immune system.

What micronutrients must the food we eat contain to keep the immune system efficient?

- Fatty acids: are the supporting structure of the cell, which is its outer layer. Viruses need a host cell to enter and multiply. For this reason, a diet rich in healthy fatty acids - such as those from avocado, dried fruits, olive oil and other oils of vegetable origin - helps to strengthen the outer layer of cells making it more difficult for viruses to access the cells.

- Antioxidants are molecules that help the organism to be defended against the attack of harmful agents and the state of oxidative stress.

The most important?

Glutathione: produced by our body, it is found in some vegetables including avocado, spinach, peaches and apples. Then there are foods capable of stimulating the production of Glutathione including those rich in Selenium such as garlic, onion, red fruits and vegetables.

Vitamin C: contained in high concentrations in all green vegetables, berries and citrus fruits; It is advisable to take this vitamin directly from fresh foods rather than from supplements because it has higher bioavailability.

Vitamin D: a deficiency of this vitamin is directly linked to an inefficient immune system; recent surveys have found a vitamin D deficiency in over 70% of the world population. Vegetable foods and in particular mushrooms are rich in it.

B-Carotene (precursor of Vitamin A): it is mainly found in carrots, pumpkin, parsley, ripe tomatoes, broccoli and green cabbage ".

There are also other micronutrients useful for keeping the immune system efficient and ready to react to external "aggressions", namely:

Selenium, Zinc and Copper, important metals for their antioxidant activity, found in legumes, mushrooms, almonds

Probiotics and prebiotics contained in all fruit and vegetables keep the microbiota healthy as they are rich in fiber.

As you may have noticed, all these elements are precisely the ones that constitute the cornerstone of an alkaline and anti-inflammatory diet.

MAKING A PLANT-BASED DIET PART OF YOUR LIFESTYLE IS EASY

HOW TO CORRECTLY BALANCE MEALS DURING THE DAY

It's easy because a plant based diet is varied and rich in foods that provide the nutrients the body needs to function at its best:

- fibers such as whole grains better if naturally poor in gluten
- proteins mostly coming from legumes
- healthy fats deriving from dried fruit
- vitamins and minerals from the many varieties of fruits and vegetables that nature offers us.

The Academy Of Nutrition and Dietetics's Journal, in 2014 published the Vegan Plate, a very useful guide that enables you to properly plan your plant nutrition in order to take all the nutrients necessary to keep us healthy. This association of nutritionists is one of the largest and most prestigious in the world and has more than 25000 members. The article is freely downloadable by anyone.

The Vegan Plate is a great graphic representation based on only vegetable foods that can ensure the correct balance of all the essential nutritional elements that our body needs. These nutritional elements are divided into six main food groups: fruits, vegetables, nuts, oilseeds, fats and proteins.

At the center of the plate, to emphasize the importance that these two vitamins have in a properly balanced plant diet, we have the nutritional elements rich in vitamin B12 and vitamin D.

It is necessary to start by quantifying one's daily caloric requirements. These requirements can change depending on if you are a male or a female, type of work and the intensity of physical activity practiced.

Once the daily caloric requirements are quantified the vegan plate must be simply equally divided into the six food categories mentioned above.

So, to know what to put in your plate without having to use scales or calorie calculations, you just have to follow the vegan plate simple and valuable indications.

In order to correctly distribute meals during the day, it is necessary to divide them in the three main meals adding 1 or 2 snacks in-between them.

An old saying says: have breakfast like a rich person, lunch like a middle-class person and dinner like a pauper.

For breakfast it is advisable to drink a good herbal tea, vegetable milk or coffee. You can prepare a porridge with whole cereal flakes, vegetable yogurt, dried fruit and chia seeds adding bitter cocoa or dark chocolate crumbles if you like. You can finish your breakfast by eating a fruit.

Snacks should include fruit – berries, having low fructose content, are excellent - or dried fruit or slices of dried coconut or high quality dark chocolate chips.

Lunch and dinner, in order to bring the right nutrients, should include, first of all, a good amount of vegetables preferably raw but also cooked or just blanched. If you start the meal with vegetables you will be able to get all the necessary enzymes to better face digestion; moreover, having vegetables a satiating power, you will tend to continue the meal without caloric exaggerations.

Lunch can also be followed by a dish of gluten free cereals - preferably whole wheat - or a dish based on vegetable proteins such as those contained in legumes.

Below is a list of cereals that do not contain gluten or contain a very digestible type of gluten such as spelt:

- Amaranth
- Black rice
- Kamut
- Quinoa
- Rya
- Emmer
- Wild rice

During the day it is recommended to drink herbal teas made by using the herbs below:

- Alvaca
- Clove
- Chamomille
- Anice
- Fennel
- Ginger
- Raspberry red
- Sea moss tea
- Lemongrass

It is also highly recommended to use spices as an ingredient to all one's dishes.

Below is a list of healthy spices and their properties:

- Curcumin - supports brain, cardiovascular and joint health, antioxidant
- Dandelion - purifier of blood and liver
- Elderberry (Sambucus nigra) - strengthens the body against colds
- Burdock root - blood and liver cleanser, diuretic,
- Bladderwrack (seaweed) - vitamins and mineral supplements
- Bromelain and papain: dissolve proteins in the small intestine
- Chlorella (seaweed) - proteins, vitamins and mineral supplements, detoxifiers
- Irish Moss (seaweed) - vitamins and mineral supplements
- Oregano oil - antiviral
- Sarsaparilla - blood purifier, antibacterial, anti-inflammatory, diuretic
- Wormwood leaf - kills parasites
- Kelp (seaweed) - vitamins and mineral supplements
- Flaxseed - fights heart disease, cancer, diabetes, high essential fatty acids

EXAMPLES OF A HEALTHY AND TASTY BREAKFAST

1) A cappuccino made with soy milk

Two slices of whole wheat spelt bread with a spread of creamy dried fruit such as hazelnuts, almonds or pistachios and thin slices of fresh fruit such as banana

2) A cup of coffee

A cup of white vegetable yogurt with cereal flakes, dried fruit such as chopped nuts and sliced fresh fruit. You can add a sprinkle of flax or chia seeds very rich in omega 3 fatty acids.

EXAMPLE OF LUNCH

Pitas topped with chickpea hummus, olive pieces and some green leafy vegetables. These vegetables are particularly rich in calcium and help those with a plant-based diet to achieve the requirements of this mineral even without consuming dairy products.

Apple slices topped with almond cream and cinnamon.

EXAMPLE OF DINNER

Quinoa with thinly sliced zucchini and boiled peas

Salad with avocado and walnuts dressed with flax seed oil.

PLANT BASED DIET AND SPORT

Sport activity doesn't just help you lose weight and sculpt your body. It's first and foremost a choice to keep us healthy.

In order to do proper sport activity it's necessary to know how to feed our body with "clean" foods that provide us with the necessary energy and that favor the recovery of the organism after having practiced sport.

Many famous sportspeople, such as Carl Lewis, have shown that they are able to achieve high-level sports performance by following a vegetable-based diet.

Those who eat a vegetable-based diet have an excellent sport performance and above all recover very quickly after sport activity.

What contributes to increase the sensation of tiredness when you practice sport is the lactic acid that the organism produces.

By following a plant-based diet the body produces less lactic acid and the lactic acid produced by the body under stress is "buffered" and disposed of more quickly because the tissues are already alkaline.

For those who do sport it's better to choose plant foods with a high protein content, such as legumes. The most protein-rich legumes are:

- soybeans

- broad beans

- lupins

Even among cereals, it is better to choose those with a higher protein content:

- oats

- amaranth

- spelt

- quinoa

- buckwheat

Finally, oilseeds and dried fruits are a real concentration of proteins: among the most protein-rich ones there are: pumpkin seeds,

- linseeds

- sesame seeds

- pine nuts

- almonds

The most famous "doping" for athletes who eat vegetables is represented by spirulina because it is rich in protein and iron.

So, there are a few tricks to increase sport performances: just know them!

HOW TO MAKE A PLANT-BASED DIET AN EMPOWERING DIET

STEP NUMBER ONE

DAILY INCLUDE THOSE FOODS THAT THE MEDICAL-SCIENTIFIC LITERATURE HAS CLASSIFIED AS SUPERFOODS.

Avocado:

A true concentration of healthy nutrients. It is rich in potassium and magnesium, mineral salts that intervene in all cellular exchanges: rich in fiber and fatty acids. The latter are easily used by our body to produce energy, avoiding insulin peaks that lead to the accumulation of body fat. Recent studies have shown how useful avocado is to prevent cancer, especially stomach and pancreatic cancer, to combat osteoporosis and to reduce the symptoms of depression.

Blueberries and red fruits:

Like all very colorful vegetables, these fruits are very rich in antioxidants that slow down cellular aging; they also have a detoxifying and anti-inflammatory function and help lower blood sugar levels; they promote the increase of healthy HDL cholesterol thus strengthening the entire cardiovascular system. Although low in sugar, they are a concentrate of flavor that should not be missing in smoothies, salads....

Cumin:

A spice with a very intense aroma that comes from a herbaceous plant from which its seeds are extracted and dried; rich in calcium, magnesium, phosphorus, vitamin A, vitamin E; great for strengthening the immune system and helps keep pathogenic viruses away.

Cinnamon:

Known all over the world for more than 2000 years; rich in phenols that slow down the putrefaction of certain foods; it is known for its aphrodisiac effect and for its ability to enhance flavors in the kitchen; regulates cholesterol levels, facilitates digestion, reduces blood glucose levels, enhances energy and even has beneficial effects on the mood.

Cabbage and broccoli:

Crucifers are very resistant to cold climates and very rich in antioxidants such as vitamin K, vitamin A, vitamin E, magnesium, omega 3 fibers, iron and potassium; a 100 grams of broccoli contain 150% of the average daily requirement of our vitamin C requirement; medical literature recognizes these plants as having a strong anti-carcinogenic power; they prevent diseases such as diabetes, osteoporosis, fortify the immune system and promote weight loss because they have the power to satiate; finally, they are rich in fibers that allow food to move faster in the intestinal tract and therefore to assimilate simple sugars less. Better to eat raw or seared in a pan.

Coconut oil:

Extracted from the fruit. Rich in MCT medium-chain triglycerides more easily used by our body to produce energy than fats of animal origin which are defined as long-chain; for this reason, when you eat coconut, its fat is immediately oxidized by the liver, immediately providing energy; therefore, it is very suitable for those who practice sports; However, it is also suitable for those who want to lose weight because on the one hand it avoids the accumulation of body fat and on the other it has strong satiating power.

It also has a strong anti-bacterial, viral, and fungal capacity thanks to the lauric acid contained in it.

Turmeric:

Is an antioxidant spice with strong free radicals and anti-cancer powers; recognized as being very important by holistic and ayurvedic medicine. Its active ingredient, curcumin, has an anti-inflammatory action, and for this reason it is used for treating arthritis, inflammation, arthrosis and joint pain. Another benefit of turmeric is that it protects the immune system.

Chocolate:

It must have a high percentage of cocoa and therefore at least 80% and possibly raw.

It is good to consume no more than 30 grams per day.

Chocolate is defined as "food of gods".

Rich in:

- magnesium
- antioxidants
- tryptophan that is an essential amino acid able to relax the nervous system and increase the quality of your sleep
- polyphenols that improves brain function and slows down cognitive decay.

- flavonoids that protect the internal wall of blood vessels, regulates blood pressure and cholesterol.

In the recipes section you can find some tasty sweets made with chocolate!

STEP NUMBER TWO

<u>INSERT DIETARY SUPPLEMENTS DAILY OR IN CYCLES</u>

To reinforce the beneficial effects of the plaint based diet, it may be advisable to supplement it with some food supplements.

Vitamin B-12

Vitamin B-12 is essential for the health of blood and neurological cells as well as for the production of DNA.

In general, people who follow vegan or vegetarian diet plans, as well as older folks, are at risk of developing B-12 deficiency.

Symptoms of B-12 deficiency include fatigue, depressed illness, tingling in the hands and feet, and anemia.

Omega-3 Essential Fatty Acids

Fundamentally, omega-3 essential fatty acids are composed of the various components of cell membranes. They aid the following areas:

- brain functioning and visual health energy
- maintaining good heart health and a good cardio circulatory system

Vitamin C or Ascorbic Acid

Although a plant based diet is rich in foods that contain vitamins it can still be important to integrate this vitamin because the cultivation soils today are less fertile than those of the past and consequently their fruits may not have the high vitamin C concentrations as they used to have.

We are also talking about a vitamin that degrades easily with heat, therefore we are not always able to assimilate it in the right quantities.

It is one of the most important vitamins because it is involved in numerous metabolic and enzymatic processes:

- Strengthens the immune defenses therefore increasing the ability of immune cells to produce antibodies; increasing the body's ability to better resist all diseases.

- It has a detoxifying effect on the body (toxins resulting from smoke or pollution).

- Protects and repairs tissues by affecting collagen production; the latter safeguards the functions of cartilage, bones, skin, capillaries and gums.

- It is antioxidant because it counteracts the negative effects of free radicals or those molecules that push our body towards premature aging

- It is useful in case of anemia because it improves the assimilation of iron which is an important mineral for the production of red blood cells.

- It helps to reduce stress by helping the synthesis of molecules that keep the transmission of nerve impulses stable; it also regulates the synthesis of the stress hormone.

Vitamin D

Our bodies are only able to synthesize vitamin D when we expose ourselves to the sun.

For those who rarely expose themselves to the sun or only at certain times of the year, it may be useful to integrate this vitamin into their diet.

This vitamin is very important:

- For the correct mineralization of bones and teeth because it helps maintain an optimal level of calico in the blood

- To help keep our kidneys, arteries and body tissues healthy

- To strengthen the system against infections and immune viruses

- To maintain the functionality of the heart and the cardio-circulatory system.

STEP NUMBER THREE

CHOOSE HIGH-QUALITY FOOD AND DON'T CONSUME FOOD THAT HAS BEEN GENETICALLY MODIFIED.

To maximize effectiveness, since it is a detox diet, it's best to buy organic or sustainable bio food and therefore not contaminated by chemicals and heavy metals.

STEP NUMBER FOUR

DRINK LOTS OF WATER, BETTER IF IT IS SPRING WATER.

Drinking plenty of water a day is important, because water is essential for a healthy and functional body; furthermore, water helps the absorption of nutrients.

It would be ideal to consume spring water.

Spring water is water that flows from rocks or from deep soils, therefore making it become a dynamic, lively and vital element.

For this reason, spring water has a full and nice taste. It quenches and refreshes us better than running water that comes out of the tap or other types of water.

In particular, if the source is alpine, the water is filtered by earthy and sandy layers which act as a filter preventing heavy pollutants from entering the water; we are therefore talking about waters that generally have excellent levels of purity.

It is also 'dynamized water', that is, water that has the ability to vitalize the body's cells and to be therapeutic for the excretory organs such as the kidneys and liver.

It is important when buying spring water to make sure that the name and location of the source, as well as the declaration of bottling at the source, are written on the bottle label.

FOOD: FIRST CURE AGAINST DISEASES

PLANT BASED DIET AND LOSING WEIGHT

We have seen how plant based diet aims to bring benefits to health, prevent serious diseases and to cure them.

But does it also make you lose weight?

As far as losing weight is concerned, even for this type of diet the principle of calorie deficit cannot be missing: no deficit no lost kilos. While it is not the motto of any diet, it is the "hidden" principle behind all weight loss eating plans.

A plant based diet was not born as a slimming diet, but in any case, following it, weight loss is the natural consequence because the foods it includes are overall not very densely caloric and are satiating as they are rich in water and dietary fiber,

The accumulated body fat, especially the one that is concentrated in the abdomen, is a first symptom of development of other diseases such as diabetes, autoimmune diseases, oncological diseases.

So it is important not to underestimate this first clue that the body gives us and act immediately to bring the metabolic system to work well.

To this end, a plant based diet helps us because:

• it contains a lot of fibers that have a satiating and satisfying effect, therefore it will pass some time before feeling the hunger stimulus

- it contains few saturated fats

PLANT BASED DIET AND NEURODEGENERATIVE DISEASE

Food, in addition to being a pleasure, is also made of chemical and biochemical molecules that interact with our cells including neurons, and can generate a favorable or unfavorable effect depending on the quality of the food we eat.

If all cells reproduce and regenerate themselves neurons are not able to do so. They are only able to regenerate and not reproduce themselves. Therefore it is better to protect them as much as possible especially after a certain age.

Certain environmentally toxic elements such as mercury, lead and heavy metals, accumulate precisely in adipose tissue and nervous tissue that has a fat component.

When inflammation becomes chronic, it can lead to the onset and development of neurodegenerative diseases such as Alzheimer's and dementia, which are becoming increasingly common: the central nervous system is made up of neurons that, if inflamed, lead to an involution of the nervous system.

Good thing is that nature always gives us its remedies. We can choose to eat those strictly vegetable foods, called "The magnificent seven" that feed and support the central nervous system.

Let's learn to use them all daily:

1. Green tea better if in the morning at breakfast

2. Ginger and turmeric better if used in the form of fresh roots

3. Dark chocolate better if processed raw, that means that cocoa beans processed to obtain chocolate must not have been submitted to a temperature higher than 42 degrees.

4. Berries which give a very abundant intake of vitamins, mineral salts and polyphenols

5. Dried fruits, except for peanuts, which are instead allergic and pro-inflammatory. Walnuts are to be preferred as they happen to resemble the shape of our brain. They are rich in omega 3 and are anti-inflammatory.

6. Oil seeds, especially flax seeds, chia seeds and hemp seeds.

7. Chlorella tea which is a freshwater alga with strong detoxifying power.

CONCLUSION

Maintaining a diet over time and then making it sustainable seems to be much more difficult than starting a diet. While most people adhere to a diet for a short period of time, that is, until they have reached their goals, what everyone finds extremely difficult is turning the diet into a new eating regime to include in their lifestyle.

One way to get us to eat healthy meals is a strategy known as "crowding out". It's quite simple: instead of eliminating bad elements from your diet, you can just include healthier foods in your diet. For example:

- you could start the meal with a certain amount of raw vegetables: this will increase satiety and alkalize the meal more;
- you can gradually incorporate new healthy eating habits: the more often you eat healthy meals, the more likely you are to get used to them and eventually start preferring them to harmful ones. It only takes a couple of weeks to turn a new habit into a habit;
- it is better to go shopping when you are not hungry: buying food when you are not full leads us to make impulse purchases and therefore not very rational purchases;
- let's remember that making a choice of vegetable food means making an ethical and eco-sustainable choice.

If our health conditions are good or if we already have pathologies, starting a vegetable-based diet can bring great benefits.

We should remember that our body is endowed with a great power: the power to heal itself.

Numerous scientific studies have led to the certainty that an adequate diet can prevent many diseases and in many cases be curative until their total remission.

However, many people are not ready to put a healthy lifestyle at the center of their daily lives. Often those who suffer from chronic illnesses are those who habitually eat foods that inflame their bodies, don't devote quality time to exercise, live under permanent stress without being able to cleanse their negative thoughts with a few minutes a day of meditation or deep relaxation.

I would like to address all these topics in more detail in another book that will be published soon.

For the moment I was happy to share with you the knowledge I have gained about clean, green, anti-inflammatory and healing nutrition.

I sincerely hope I was able to make you more aware of how much we can increase the quality of our lives by simply "eating" not only what is readily available, but what we have chosen with conscience and awareness.

Good continuation of your personal journey into a more and more "conscious" nutrition!

RECIPES

The following recipes are a selection of dishes easy to prepare demonstrating that healthy food can be good and also be very tasty.

And now.................Bon appetite!

LASAGNA WITH CARASAU BREAD

Time required for preparation: 20 minutes

Cooking time: 20 minutes

Serving: 4

Ingredients:
- 200 g carasau bread or pitas bread
- 700 ml soy milk
- 40 g of almond flour
- 400 g of spinach
- 70 g of spelt flour
- Salt
- Pepper
- Nutmeg
- Extra virgin olive oil

Preparation:
1. Boil the spinach and drain well from the water and let it cool.
2. In another pot combine the flour and soy milk stirring with a whisk to mix well
3. Add salt, pepper and nutmeg.
4. Bring the béchamel sauce to a boil over low heat, stirring until creamy. Allow to cool.
5. Add two tablespoons of oil and the spinach.
6. Take a casserole dish and form the layers of lasagna alternating the spinach cream with carasau bread

slightly moistened with a little water or soy milk. Between each layer add the almond flour.

Finish with a slice of corasau bread. Add a little oil before placing in preheated oven at 200 degrees for 20 minutes.

Nutrition
- Calories in a serving: 350
- 4 g of fat
- Carbohydrates: 59 g
- 19 g of protein

AVOCADO, TOFU AND ASPARAGUS TARTARE

Time required for preparation: 20 minutes

Cooking time: 10 minutes

Serving: 2

Ingredients:
- 250 g asparagus
- 80 g tofu cut into cubes
- 1 lime
- 4 tablespoons of extra virgin olive oil 40
- A handful of toasted pine nuts
- A pinch of ground mustard
- Salt and pepper
- A pinch of garlic powder
- Fresh Basil

Preparation:
1. Cook the asparagus for 10 minutes.
2. Emulsify oil, garlic, juice of half a lime, basil and mustard powder.
3. Dice the avocado and drizzle the remaining lime juice over it so it doesn't darken.
4. Season chopped asparagus, avocado and tofu in a large bowl with the oil emulsion.
5. Prepare the tartare by pouring half of the compost into a ramekin previously placed in the center of the plate.

6. Garnish with toasted pine nuts.

Nutrition

- Calories in a serving: 440
- 35 g of fat
- Carbohydrates: 5,9 g
- 18 g of protein

FLAXSEED CRACKERS

Time required for preparation: 20 minutes

Cooking time: 10 minutes

Serving: 6

Ingredients:

- 200 g millet or spelt flour
- 35 g of extra virgin olive oil
- a pinch of dried chives
- 60 g of flax seeds
- 200 ml of water
- a pinch of salt

Preparation:

1. Put all the ingredients in a large bowl, mix everything with your hands until you get a homogeneous dough.
2. Give the dough the shape of a ball, wrap it in plastic wrap and refrigerate for about two hours.
3. Heat the oven to 200 degrees.
4. Roll out the dough on baking paper and give it the shape of a rectangle with a fairly thin thickness.
5. Place the dough in an oven dish and with a knife cut it into squares the size of crackers.
6. Bake for about ten minutes.
7. Remove from the oven and allow the crackers to cool before removing them from each other.

Nutrition

- Calories in a serving: 195
- 11 g of fat

- Carbohydrates: 20 g
- 11 g of protein

CABBAGE ROLL CASSEROLE WITH A TWIST

Time required for preparation: 10 minutes

Cooking time: 40 minutes

Serving: 4

Ingredients:

- 1 cup cooked of quinoa
- One and a half red onions
- Finely chopped 2 garlic cloves,
- Minced four white mushrooms,
- Finely chopped one and a half cans of diced tomatoes,
- Vegetable stock or homemade vegetable broth
- 1 cup of fresh basil leaves, minced
- 8 green cabbage leaves, whole
- 2 teaspoons of extra virgin olive oil

Instructions:

1. Turn on the oven and set it to a temperature of 350 degrees Fahrenheit.
2. In a non-stick pan, add the extra virgin olive oil, the onion, quinoa, garlic clove, and chopped the onion, quinoa, garlic clove, and chopped mushrooms. Cook for 5 minutes. Add the tomato sauce, vegetable stock, and basil. Mix well. Continue to cook for another 10 minutes.

3. Place 2 cabbage leaves on top of the baking sheet. Put a quarter of the filling on top, close the cabbage leaves with kitchen twine. Repeat to make the other three rolls.
4. Bake in the oven for 40 minutes covered with aluminum foil.
5. Allow for a 10-minute resting period before serving.

Nutrition

- Calories in a serving: 261
- 2 g of fat
- Carbohydrates: 51 g
- 12 g of protein

CASSEROLE WITH MANGO, QUINOA AND NLACK BEANS AND TANGY SAUCE

Time required for preparation: 10 minutes

Cooking time: 25 minutes

Servings: 4

Ingredients:

- 2 cups of coconut milk
- 1 cup vegetable stock or homemade vegetable broth
- 2 cups of cooked quinoa
- Drain and rinse 2 cups of black beans before using
- 1/4 cup of minced fresh mint
- 1 mango peeled and cut
- 1 avocado peeled and cut
- A pinch of Himalayan pink salt
- 2 teaspoons of extra virgin olive oil

Instructions:

1. Preheat the oven to 425 degrees Fahrenheit.
2. Place the stock, milk, and quinoa in a casserole dish and mix well.
3. Bake for 25 minutes, covered with aluminum foil.
4. Turn off the oven and remove the baking dish. Combine the beans, mango, avocado and fresh mint in a large mixing bowl.

5. Finish by seasoning with salt and oil and serving.

Nutrition

- 573 calories in a serving
- 23 g of fat
- Carbohydrates: 75 g
- 15 g of protein

PEPPERS AND ONIONS MASALA

Time required for preparation: 10 minutes

Cooking preparation: 30 minutes

Serving: 2

Ingredients:

- 1 cup of uncooked brown rice
- 2 tablespoons of coconut oil
- 1 tbsp. of ground cumin seeds
- 1/2 teaspoon of freshly ground turmeric
- 2 onions, peeled and finely chopped
- 2 green chilies, finely diced (1-inch)
- 1 piece of fresh ginger
- 2 grated garlic cloves
- 2 tablespoons of extra virgin olive oil
- 3 tablespoons of tomato paste
- 1 teaspoon of chilli powder
- A pinch of Himalayan pink salt.
- Washed and sliced 1 red bell pepper

Instructions:

1. Place the brown rice in a small saucepan with enough boiling water to cover it over medium-low heat and cook for 25 to 30 minutes, or until the rice is done.

2. In the meanwhile, heat the coconut oil in a nonstick skillet. Add the cumin seeds, turmeric, onion, garlic, chili, and ginger. Cook for 5 minutes.
3. Stir in the tomato paste and chili powder and add salt. Make a thorough mix.
4. Cook for another 5 minutes once you've added the bell pepper
5. Toss the rice with the hot masala and serve immediately.
6. Dress with extra virgin olive oil

Nutrition

- Calories in a serving: 520
- Carbohydrates: 81 g
- 8 g fat
- 6 g of dietary fiber
- 4 g of sugar
- 4 g of protein

PIZZA WITH BASIL AND OLIVES

Time required for preparation: 10 minutes

Cooking preparation: 30 minutes

Servings: 4

Ingredients:

For the pizza sauce, use the following ingredients:

- 1 (15-ounce) can of diced tomatoes
- 1 tablespoon extra-virgin olive oil
- 1/2 cup fresh basil leaves, rinsed thoroughly
- 2 garlic cloves, peeled and chopped
- 1 teaspoon of onion powder
- 1/4 teaspoon dried sage
- Red chilli flakes (1/4 teaspoon) (optional)
- 1 teaspoon of pink Himalayan salt

For the pizza, use the following ingredients:

- 4 pitas bread made with permitted flours
- Shredded vegan mozzarella (4 ounces).
- Rinse and thinly slice 1 cup mixed vegetables of your choice (tomatoes; eggplant; onion; green pepper; mushroom)
- 1/3 cup pitted olives, finely chopped
- 1 tablespoon extra-virgin olive oil
- 5 basil leaves, washed and split into tiny pieces

Instructions:

To prepare the sauce, follow these steps:

1. In a blender, blend on low speed until the basil and garlic are very tiny bits, then add the olive oil and blend until smooth.
2. Put diced tomatoes, the onion powder, the salt and cook for about 20 minutes, or until the sauce has reduced somewhat and thickened in a saucepan.

To prepare the pizza, follow these steps:

1. Set the oven to 500 degrees Fahrenheit. Prepare a baking sheet by lining it with parchment paper and setting it aside.
2. Spread the pizza sauce over the pitas in a uniform layer. Place the vegan mozzarella on top and sprinkle the cut vegetables and olives, the basil and garlic emulsion and dried sage.
3. Bake for about 8 minutes.
4. Drizzle the pizzas with olive oil and sprinkle the basil leaves on top of them to finish. For about three weeks, you can store leftovers in the freezer in an airtight container.

Nutrition

- Calories in a serving: 400
- 10 g of total fat
- Carbohydrates: 64 g
- 5 g of dietary fiber
- 2 g of sugar

- 10 g of protein

BLACK BEAN CHILI

Time for preparation: 15 minutes

Cooking time: 20 minutes

Serving: 2

Ingredients:

- 1 tablespoon of coconut oil
- 1 medium-sized onion, peeled and chopped
- 6 mushrooms, cleaned and cut into slices
- 2 tablespoons of freshly ground coriander
- 2 tablespoons of paprika
- 2 tbsp. of cumin seeds
- 1 tablespoon of freshly grated nutmeg
- 1 tablespoon of chilli powder
- 1 (15-ounce) can of diced tomatoes
- 1 can of rinsed black beans
- 1 can of rinsed kidney beans
- 5 cherry tomatoes, drained and rinsed
- 2 tablespoons of tomato purée
- 7 oz. of uncooked brown rice (optional)
- 4 tablespoons of coconut yoghurt, to be used for serving (optional)
- 4 fresh cilantro sprigs, to be used for garnishing (optional)

Instructions:

1. Place the coconut oil over medium heat in a large skillet. Add the onion and cook for two minutes then add the mushrooms and cook for another 4 minutes. Combine the coriander, paprika, cumin, cinnamon and chilli powder until well combined.
2. Stir in the canned tomatoes and their juices, black beans, kidney beans, cherry tomatoes, and tomato purée until everything is well-combined. All ingredients should be stirred together and brought to a simmer. Cook for 25 minutes at medium heat.
3. While the chilli is cooking, prepare the rice according to the directions on the box. Drain after rinsing.
4. Arrange the chilli on top of the rice, topped with yoghurt (if using) and cilantro, and serve immediately (if using).

Nutrition

- Calories in a serving: 580
- 5 g of total fat
- Carbohydrates: 102 g
- 18 g of dietary fibre
- 14 g of sugar
- 19 g of protein

LENTILS IN A VARIETY OF COLORS

Time required for preparation: 15 minutes

Cooking preparation: 30 minutes

Servings: 4

Ingredients:

- 2 tablespoons of coconut oil
- 1 onion, peeled
- 2 carrots that have been peeled and chopped
- 2 celery stalks, washed and chopped
- 1 sweet potato, washed and chopped
- 1 cup cooked lentils
- 5 cups vegetable stock
- To taste, add a pinch of Himalayan pink salt

Instructions:

1. Over medium heat, heat the coconut oil until it shimmers. Add the onion and cook for 3 minutes.
2. Add the carrots, celery and sweet potato to the remaining ingredients and continue cooking for another 2 minutes.
3. Pour in the lentils and the vegetable stock. Stir constantly until the lentils are tender, about 25 minutes.
4. Season to taste with salt before serving.

Nutrition

- Calories in a serving: 330
- Carbs: 49 g
- Fat: 10 g
- 20 g of fiber
- 8 g of sugar
- 17 g of protein

PASTA WITH TOMATOES AND SPELT

Time required for preparation: 15 minutes

Cooking time: 20 minutes

Servings: 4

Ingredients:

- Extra-virgin olive oil (around 3 tablespoons)
- 2 garlic cloves, peeled and smashed
- 1 diced onion
- 1 eggplant (rinsed and chopped)
- 2 zucchinis, peeled and diced
- 2 or 3 tomatoes, washed and chopped
- 1 cup of sun-dried tomatoes
- 2 tsp dried basil (optional)
- 1 tablespoon dried oregano leaves
- 1 tbsp. wine vinegar
- A pinch of Himalayan pink salt
- 7 ounces of spelt pasta

Instructions:

1. Over medium heat, shimmer the olive oil in a large skillet. Sauté the garlic, onion, and eggplant for 8 minutes, or until the eggplant is soft.
2. Combine the zucchini, tomatoes, sun-dried tomatoes, basil, and oregano in a large mixing bowl. Cook for 8 minutes, stirring occasionally. Season with salt.

3. Place the pasta in a separate pot with enough boiling water to cover it and simmer for approximately 10 minutes, or until the pasta is tender but not falling apart.
4. Serve the pasta immediately with the sauce.

Nutrition

- Calories: 460 per serving
- 12 g of total fat
- Carbohydrates: 75 g
- 17 g of protein
- 11 g of sugar

CRISPY GREEN TOMATOES ON A STICK

Time required for preparation: 14 minutes

Cooking time: 16 minutes

Servings: 2

Ingredients:

- 1/4 cup of coconut flour
- Pinch of salt
- 4 sliced green tomatoes
- 1 cup of homemade applesauce
- 1/2 cup of almond flour
- 1/4 cup of extra-virgin olive oil

Instructions:

1. To begin, combine the coconut flour, salt in a large mixing basin. Toss the tomatoes together. Toss until everything is thoroughly covered.
2. Pour the apple sauce into a separate mixing dish. Toss in the almond flour. Combine until everything is well-combined.
3. Bring the oil to a boil. Dip the tomatoes into the apple sauce mixture. Repeat with the remaining tomatoes. Using batches, fry the tomatoes for about 3 minutes each until golden brown. Serve.

Nutrition

- Calories in a serving: 113
- Fat: 4.2 g
- Saturated fat: 0.8 g
- Cholesterol: 0 milligram
- Sodium: 861 milligram
- Carbohydrates: 22.5 g
- Fiber: 6.3 g
- Sugar: 2.3 g
- Protein: 9.2 g

FRUIT SALAD IN CIDER

Time required for preparation: 11 minutes

Cooking time: 16 minutes

Servings: 3

Ingredients:

- 1 small apple, cubed
- 1 small apricot, cubed
- Grapefruit pulp, shredded into bite-sized pieces
- 1/4 cup jacamar, cubed
- 2 tablespoons apple cider vinegar, warmed in the microwave
- 1 tablespoon of cider sauce
- A pinch of ground cinnamon powder

Instructions:

1. Whisk together the apple cider vinegar and cinnamon powder in a small mixing basin.
2. The salad ingredients should be combined in a large mixing bowl with the cider sauce, the apple cider vinegar and cinnamon. Toss everything together well; divide the mixture among the dishes in equal quantities. Serve as soon as possible.

Nutrition

- 123 calories per serving
- Fats: 14.2 g

- Saturated fat: 0.7 g
- Total fat: 14.2 g
- Cholesterol: 0 milligram
- Sodium: 661 milligram
- Carbohydrates: 22.5 g
- 6.3 g of dietary fiber
- 0 g of sugar
- 9.2 gram of protein

STIR-FRY WITH ZUCCHINI AND BROCCOLI

Time required for preparation: 15 minutes

Cooking time: 15 minutes

Serving: 4

Ingredients:

- Coconut oil and sesame oil, 2 tablespoons each
- 1 piece of fresh ginger, peeled and finely chopped
- 4 garlic cloves, peeled and minced
- 2 onions (rinsed and chopped)
- 1 broccoli head, washed and split into florets
- 1-cup of steamed zucchini, washed and sliced into long
- 3-scallions peeled and finely chopped
- 1 tablespoon finely chopped fresh basil leaves
- 1-ounce coconut amino acid

Instructions:

1. Heat the coconut and sesame oils in a wok or big pan over medium heat. Add the ginger and garlic. Cook for 5 minutes.
2. Add the onions and broccoli to the pan and simmer for 3 minutes, or until the onion begins to soften a little.

3. Combine the zucchini, scallions, and basil. Toss everything together and cook for 4 minutes until the veggies are soft and delicious.
4. Turn off the heat, sprinkle in the coconut amino, and transfer to a serving platter.

Nutrition

- Calories in a serving: 180
- 14 g of total fat
- Carbohydrates: 13 g
- 3 g of dietary fiber
- 4 g of sugar
- 3 g of protein

KAMUT NOODLES WITH PESTO

Time required for preparation: 5 minutes

Cooking time: 15 minutes

Servings: 2

Ingredients:

- Extra-virgin olive oil (around 3 tablespoons)
- 1 bunch of freshly picked basil leaves
- 6 cups of well washed cooked kamut noodles (cooked according to package directions)
- 1 bunch of fresh parsley
- 1 bunch of fresh cilantro
- A pinch of Himalayan pink salt

Instructions:

1. Combine the olive oil, basil, parsley, and cilantro in a blender until well combined. Blend until the mixture is smooth.
2. Combine the cooked noodles and the sauce in a large mixing basin. Toss to combine flavours.

Nutrition

- Calories in a serving: 355
- Total fat: 21
- Carbohydrates: 36 g
- Dietary fiber: 1 g
- Protein: 9 g

QUINOA BOWL

Time required for preparation: 10 minutes

Time required for cooking: 10 minutes

Servings: 4

Ingredients:

- 1 cup of quinoa, well washed
- 1 cup of water brought to a boil
- 1 can of rinsed black beans
- One teaspoon of cumin seeds,
- 2 minced garlic cloves,
- 2 limes (squeezed)
- Avocado thinly sliced
- Fresh cilantro (about one handful)

Instructions:

1. Pour the quinoa inside the boiling water and mix. Cook it for about 8 minutes.
2. While that's happening, in a small skillet combine the black beans, scallions, garlic, cumin and lime juice.
3. Simmer for 10 minutes.
4. Combine the quinoa and warmed beans in a large mixing basin until well combined. Place the avocado and cilantro over the top and serve immediately.

Nutrition

- 420 calories per serving
- 9 g of total fat
- Carbohydrates: 70 g
- 18 g of dietary fibre
- 2 g of sugar
- 10 g of protein

ROASTED VEGETABLES

Time required for preparation: 14 minutes

Cooking time: 17 minutes

Servings: 2

Ingredients:

- 2 cups of olive oil,
- 2 heads of big garlic
- 2 big eggplants
- 2 large shallots peeled, then quartered
- 2 carrots, peeled and cut into cubes
- 1 giant parsnip, peeled and cut into cubes
- 1 small green bell pepper
- 1 broccoli
- 1 big sprig of thyme, with leaves plucked
- A pinch of salt

Ingredients for garnishing

- ½ lemon divided into wedges and ½ squeezed
- 1 / 8 cup fennel bulb, finely chopped

Instructions:

1. Preheat the oven until the temperature reaches 425 degrees Fahrenheit.

2. Prepare a deep roasting pan by lining it with aluminum foil and gently greasing it with oil. Toss in all the vegetables, herbs and salt to taste.
3. Add the remaining oil and lemon juice until well combined. Toss everything together well.
4. To cover the roasting pan, place a piece of aluminum foil. Place this on the center oven rack and bake for 30 minutes. Remove the aluminum foil from the pan. After cooling for a few minutes, divide evenly among plates.
5. Finish with a fennel bulb, finely chopped and a slice of lemon for garnish. Before you begin to eat, squeeze the lemon juice over the top of the meal.

Nutrition

- Calories in a serving: 164
- Fat: 4.2 g
- Saturated fat: 0.8 g
- Cholesterol: 0 milligrams
- Sodium: 861 milligrams
- Carbohydrates: 22.5 g
- 6.3 g of dietary fiber
- Sugar: 23 g
- 9.2 grams of protein

PILAF EMMER

Time required for preparation: 10 minutes

Cooking time: 15 minutes

Servings: 4

Ingredients:

- 1 cup of emmer
- filtered water
- 4 cleaned, seeded, and chopped tomatoes
- Extra-virgin olive oil (around 2 tablespoons)
- 1/4 cup of chopped dried apricot
- 1 teaspoon grated lemon zest
- 1 tbsp. lemon juice
- 1/2 cup of finely chopped fresh parsley (rinsed and chopped)
- A pinch of Himalayan pink salt

Instructions:

1. Place the emmer and tomatoes in a pot full of water. Boil for 15 minutes and drain.
2. Combine the olive oil, apricots, lemon zest, lemon juice, and parsley in a large mixing bowl. Adjust seasonings if needed, and serve.

Nutrition

- Calories in a serving: 270

- Fat: 8 g
- Carbohydrates: 42 g
- 5 g of dietary fiber
- 3 g of sugar
- 6 g of protein

ONIONS WITH A SWEET AND SOUR TASTE

Time required for preparation: 10 minutes

Cooking time: 11 minutes

Servings: 4

Ingredients:

- A vegetable stock or homemade vegetable broth
- 6 big onions halved
- 2 garlic cloves crushed
- 1/2 tablespoon of balsamic vinegar
- 1/2 teaspoon of Dijon mustard
- 1 tablespoon agave syrup

Instructions:

1. In a large skillet, combine the onions and garlic. Fry for 3 minutes or until the vegetables are tender.
2. Combine the stock, vinegar, Dijon mustard, and agave syrup.
3. Make sure the heat is turned down. Simmer the mixture under a cover for 10 minutes.
4. Remove yourself from the heat. Continue stirring after the liquid has been reduced and the onions have become brown. Serve.

Nutrition

- 203 calories per serving
- Fat: 41.2 g
- Saturated Fat: 0.8 g
- Sodium: 861 milligrams
- Carbohydrates: 29.5 g
- 16.3 g of dietary fiber
- 29.3 g of sugar
- 19.2 grams of protein

APPLES AND ONIONS SAUTÉED WITH OLIVE OIL

Time required for preparation: 14 minutes

Cooking time: 16 minutes

Servings: 2

Ingredients:

- 2 cups of unsweetened apple cider
- 1 big onion, peeled and halved
- A vegetable stock
- 4 apples, peeled and cut into wedges
- A pinch of sea salt

Instructions:

1. In a medium-sized pot, combine the cider and onion. Cook until the onions are soft and the liquid has dried.
2. Put in the stock and apples, seasoning with salt to taste Cook them for approximately 10 minutes. Serve.

Nutrition

- Calories in a serving : 343
- Total fat: 50.12 g
- Saturated fat: 0.8 g
- Cholesterol: 0 milligrams

- Sodium: 861 milligrams
- Carbohydrates: 22.5 g
- 6.3 g of dietary fiber
- 2.3 g of sugar
- 9.2 g of protein

ZUCCHINI NOODLES WITH PORTOBELLO MUSHROOMS

Time required for preparation: 14 minutes

Cooking time: 16 minutes

Servings: 2

Ingredients:

- 1 zucchini, shredded and made into spaghetti-like strands
- 3 garlic cloves, peeled and minced
- 2 finely sliced white onions (optional)
- 1 inch of julienned ginger
- 2 pounds of portobello mushrooms, cut into thick slivers
- Pinch of sea salt
- 2 table spoons of sesame oil
- 2 tablespoons of coconut oil
- 1/4 cup finely chopped fresh chives (for garnish)

Instructions:

1. Melt 2 tablespoons of coconut oil over medium heat in a saucepan. Cook mushroom slivers for 5 minutes or until brown.
2. Add the onion, garlic, and ginger and cook for three minutes, until the onion is soft.
3. Bring the water to a boil. Reduce the heat gradually and allow the zucchini to simmer for 1

minute, drain and add the onion and mushroom sauce and sesame oil.

4. To serve, divide the zucchini noodles into equal portions and arrange them in individual dishes. Top the dish with chives.

Nutrition

- 163 calories in a serving
- Saturated fat is present: 0.8 g
- Cholesterol: 0 milligrams
- Sodium: 861 milligrams
- Carbohydrates: 22.5 g
- 6.3 g of dietary fiber
- 0 g of sugar
- 4.2 grams of protein

TEMPEH WITH PINEAPPLE ON THE GRILL

Time required for preparation: 12 minutes

Cooking time: 16 minutes

Servings: 2

Ingredients:

- 1 package tempeh (10 ounces, sliced)
- 1/4 pineapple, cut into rings
- 1 tablespoon of coconut oil
- Orange juice (about 2 tablespoons, freshly squeezed),
- Freshly squeezed lemon juice (about 1 tablespoon),
- 1 tablespoon of extra virgin olive oil

Instructions:

1. Combine the olive oil, orange and lemon juice and coconut oil in a large mixing bowl until well combined. Put the tempeh to marinate in the bowl for e few minutes.
2. Heat a grill pan over medium-high heat until hot. Lift the marinated tempeh out of the bowl with a pair of tongs and place it on the grill pan after it has reached a high temperature.
3. Grill for 2 to 3 minutes.
4. Slice the pineapples, grill it for a few minutes and place them on a serving plate.

5. Place the grilled tempeh and pineapple on a serving tray. Serve as soon as possible.

Nutrition

- 163 calories per serving
- Saturated fat is present: 0.8 g
- Cholesterol: 0 milligrams
- Sodium: 861 milligrams
- Carbohydrates: 22.5 g
- 6.3 g of dietary fiber
- 0 g of sugar
- 9.2 grams of protein

COURGETTES WITH APPLE CIDER SAUCE

Time required for preparation: 10 minutes

Cooking time: 17 minutes

Servings: 2

Ingredients:

- 2 cups of baby courgettes (cut in half)
- 3 tbsp. of vegetable stock (optional)
- 2 tbsp. of apple cider vinegar (optional)
- 1 tablespoon light brown sugar (optional)
- Onions, thinly cut (about 4)
- A piece of grated ginger root (fresh or dried)
- 1 tablespoon of quinoa flour
- 2 teaspoons of water

Instructions:

1. To begin grill the courgette slices
2. While that's going on, in a saucepan, add the vegetable stock, apple cider vinegar, brown sugar, onions, ginger root. Bring the mixture to a boil. Reduce the heat to low and allow for 3 minutes of simmering.
3. Combine the quinoa flour and water in a mixing bowl. Make a thorough stir. Pour the sauce into the saucepan.
4. Put the courgettes in a serving dish. Add the onion source and le quinoa cream over the top.

Nutrition

- Calories: 173 per serving
- 9.2 g of total fat
- Saturated fat is present: 0.8 g
- Cholesterol: 0 milligrams
- Sodium: 861 milligrams
- Carbohydrates: 22.5 g
- Fiber: 6.3
- Sugar: 2.3 g
- 9.2 grams of protein

BAKED MIXED MUSHROOMS

Time required for preparation: 8 minutes

Cooking time: 20 minutes

Servings: 2

Ingredients:

- 2 cups of mixed mushrooms
- 2 shallots
- 2 garlic cloves
- 3 cups of toasted chopped pecans
- 2 sprigs of fresh thyme
- 1 bunch of flat-leaf parsley
- 2 tablespoons of extra-virgin olive oil
- 2 bay leaves
- 1/2 cup of stale spelled bread

Instructions:

1. Finely chop the garlic once it has been peeled.
2. Chop the mixed mushrooms into small pieces. Wash them well. Pick the thyme leaves and tear the bread into tiny pieces with your fingers.
3. Pick the parsley leaves and coarsely chop them in a bowl.
4. Cook it for 12 minutes shallots, mixed mushrooms, oil and garlic. Add thyme, bay leaves and adjust the flavor as needed. Cook another 5 minutes.
5. Transfer the mushroom mixture to a 20 cm by 25 cm baking dish that has been covered with aluminum foil.
6. Add pecans and parsley on the top.

7. Bake for 35 minutes at 350°F in the oven. After that, remove the foil and continue to cook for another 10 minutes. Serve the finished dish with toast spelled bread.

Nutrition

- Calories in a serving: 343
- Total fat: 4.3
- Saturated fat: 0.8 g
- Cholesterol: 0 milligrams
- Sodium: 861 milligrams
- Carbohydrates: 22.5 g
- 6.3 g of fiber,
- Sugar: 2.3
- 9.2 grams of protein

OKRA WITH A SPICY TWIST

Time required for preparation: 14 minutes

Cooking time: 16 minutes

Servings: 2

Ingredients:

- 2 cups of okra
- 1/2 tbsp. of freshly ground turmeric
- 2 tablespoons of finely chopped fresh coriander
- 1 tablespoon of cumin seeds, ground
- 1/4 tbsp. of salt
- 1 tablespoon of desiccated coconut
- 3 tablespoons of extra virgin olive oil
- 1/2 teaspoons of black mustard seeds
- 1/2 teaspoon of cumin seeds
- 1 teaspoon of coconut oil
- To finish it off, 2 fresh tomatoes

Instructions:

1. Trim the okra to the desired length. Rinse and dry thoroughly.
2. Mix turmeric, fresh coriander, cumin, salt, and desiccated coconut until well combined.
3. Make sure the mustard and cumin seeds are fragrant by cooking them in a skillet for 3 minutes with coconut oil. Add the okra. Add the spice mixture. Cook for 8 minutes on a low heat setting.
4. Transfer the mixture to a serving plate. Garnish with sliced fresh tomatoes if desired.

Nutrition

- Calories in a serving 183
- 4 g fats,
- 0.8 g saturated fat
- Cholesterol: 0 milligram's
- Sodium: 861 milligrams Carbohydrates: 22.5 g
- Fiber: 6.3 g
- Sugar: 2.3 g
- Protein: 9.2 g

GREEN SOUP WITH ALKALIZING PROPERTIES

Time required for preparation: 10 minutes

Cooking: 10 minutes

servings: 2

Ingredients:

- A tbsp. of coconut oil
- 1 pint of stock
- 2 sweets potatoes
- 1/4 teaspoon of fennel seeds
- one and a half red onions
- 2 broccoli
- 4 cups baby spinach (drained)
- 1 tablespoon of lemon juice and zest
- 1 garlic clove, peeled and coarsely chopped

Instructions:

1. In a bit of oil, fry the garlic, red onions, and fennel seeds for approximately 2 minutes over medium heat.
2. Add the broccoli, lemon zest, stock, and lemon juice and simmer for 4 minutes, stirring occasionally.
3. When the spinach has wilted, remove the pan from the stove.
4. Immediately transfer the contents to a blender and process until completely smooth and creamy.

Nutrition

- Calories in a serving: 218
- 7.2 g of fat
- Saturated fat:3.8 g
- 3 milligrams of cholesterol
- Sodium: 801-milligram
- Carbohydrates: 12.5 g
- Fiber: 3.3 g

SOUP WITH GINGER AND CARROTS

Time required for preparation: 10 minutes

Cooking time: 15 minutes

Servings: 2

Ingredients:

- 1 tablespoon of grated fresh ginger
- 1/2 tablespoon of salt
- 2 garlic cloves
- quarter onion
- 4 carrots, peeled and cut into chunks
- 2 liters of vegetarian broth
- 1 teaspoon of turmeric

Instructions:

1. Stir together all the ingredients, and bring to a boil for an hour.
2. Let it cool down.
3. Mix them with an immersion blender until you get a smooth and creamy mixture.
4. If desired, sprinkle some hemp seeds on top of the dish as a garnish.

Nutrition

- Calories in 210 per serving
- 8.2 g of fat
- Saturated fat:3.8 g
- 2 milligrams of cholesterol

- Sodium: 801-milligram
- Carbohydrates: 12.5 g
- Fiber: 5.3 g

SALAD DE KALE

Time required for preparation: 10 minutes

Cooking time: 5 minutes

servings: 2

Ingredients:

- 1 avocado cut into slices
- 1 head of kale, washed, dried and thinly sliced
- 1 medium tomato

For Dressings

- 2 tablespoons of extra-virgin olive oil
- 1 teaspoon of Dijon mustard (optional)
- 4 drops of liquid stevia extract
- 1 tbsp. of lemon juice

Garnishes include:

- A few pumpkin seeds
- A few pieces of tempeh that have been seared

Instructions:

1. In a bowl, mix together all the dressing ingredients and use them to dress the kale.
2. Put in a salad bowl the avocado and the kale.
3. Season and serve with garnishes.

Nutrition

- Calories in a serving: 248
- Fat: 4.2 g
- Saturated fat: 2.8 g
- Cholesterol: 0.5 milligrams (mg)
- Sodium: 813 milligrams
- Carbohydrates: 13.5 g
- Fiber: 3.3 g

CURRY WITH TURMERIC AND ROASTED CAULIFLOWER

Time required for preparation: 10 minutes

Cooking time: 35 minutes

Servings: 4

Before beginning, it is essential to understand that this meal contains four of the most effective anti-inflammatory substances available and that is: bell pepper, turmeric, ginger, and garlic.

This meal also contains healthy fats that derive from coconut oil, seeds and almonds. So when you consume this meal you can be sure that you are ensuring an excellent service for your body's immune system.

Ingredients:

- Turmeric powder (about 1 teaspoon)
- 1 and a half cups of water
- 1 teaspoon of Himalayan salt
- 1/2 teaspoons of chili powder
- 2 florets of cauliflower cut into slices
- 1 tablespoon of coriander, finely chopped
- Unsweetened coconut milk (about 2 cups)
- 2 tablespoons of coconut oil
- 1 garlic clove, peeled and minced
- 1 teaspoon of ginger powder
- 1/2 cup of almonds

Instructions:

1. Pre-heat the oven to 400 °F.
2. Mix the almonds, the spices, water, coconut milk, coconut oil, a teaspoon of salt, and cauliflower.
3. Using your hands, thoroughly combine the ingredients.
4. Get out a baking pan and pour in the mixture.
5. Cook in the oven for 30 minutes.

Nutrition

- Calories in a serving : 263
- Fat: 4.2
- Saturated fat :4.2
- Cholesterol 1.5 milligrams
- Sodium: 843 milligrams
- Carbohydrates: 12.5 g
- Fiber: 2.3 g

TORTILLA SOUP WITH A SPRING WATER

Time required for preparation: 15 minutes

Cooking time: 10 minutes

Servings: 4

Tortilla soup is a visually appealing combination of nutritious and alkalized food products woven together to create a flavorful and spicy meal.

Ingredients:

- 1 ripe avocado cut into slices
- 500 milliliters of spring water
- 1/2 tablespoon of coriander
- 4 handfuls of spinach
- 4 tortillas
- A pinch of Himalayan salt
- 1 teaspoon of cumin
- 2 tablespoons of extra virgin olive oil

Instructions:

1. Cut your tortilla into strips 5 cm long and 1 cm wide, and gently toast them on a hot grill.
2. Prepare the vegetable broth using spring water

3. Add the spinach, cumin and a pinch of salt to the broth. Cook for 10 minutes, turn off the heat and let it cool.
4. Place the soup on the plates and garnish with the tortilla slices, avocado and extra virgin olive oil.

Nutrition

- 157 calories in a serving
- Fat: 7.2
- Saturated fat:4.8
- Cholesterol 2.5 milligrams
- Sodium: 843 milligrams
- Carbohydrates: 12.5 g
- Fiber: 2.3 g

MINESTRONE SOUP WITH A KICK

Time required for preparation: 15 minutes

Cooking time: 15 minutes

Servings: 2

The "Hearty Minestrone" is packed with alkaline nutrients and it is also unbelievably delicious. By preparing it you simply perform an excellent service for your body. This vegetable minestrone is a good source of minerals and fiber; it also contains various vitamins and phytonutrients, which act as antioxidants.

The mix of carrots, zucchini, and sweet potatoes contained in this dish leaves no question to the fact that it is tasty, nutritious, and healthful.

Ingredients:

- 1 bunch of basil
- 1 carrot
- 2 cups of mashed sweet potato
- 1 red onion
- 1 tablespoon of coconut oil
- 1 liter of vegetable broth
- 1 cup of tomato juice
- 1/2 cup of cooked beans
- Black pepper and Himalayan salt

Instructions:

1. Peel and dice the onion, the carrot and the zucchini.
2. For 2 minutes, heat the oil in a large pan and fry the onion, carrot and zucchini.
4. Stir in the tomato juice, stock, and beans until well combined.
5. Bring the mixture to a boil, add the mashed sweet potato and decrease the heat to a low level; cook for 8–10 minutes.
6. Stir in the basil and add salt and pepper.

Nutrition

- Calories in a serving: 110
- Fat: 6.4 g
- Saturated fat: 2.8 g
- Carbohydrates: 11.3 g
- Fiber: 3.5 g

ZUCCHINI NOODLES SERVED RAW

Time required for preparation: 15 minutes

Cooking time: 10 minutes

Servings: 2

Ingredients:

- 3 medium-sized zucchinis
- Chopped spring onions
- Coconut oil (three tablespoons)
- 1 bunch coriander freshly chopped (about 1 tablespoon)

To make the sauce

- A piece of grated ginger root
- 1/4 cup of tamari and 1/4 cup tahini
- 2 teaspoons of lemon or lime juice
- 1/4 cup of almond butter
- 1 garlic clove, peeled and minced
- 1 tablespoon of coconut sugar

Instructions:

1. Begin with the courgette and carrot noodles, which should be sliced thinly using a mandolin or vegetable peeler.
2. For the sauce, combine the grated ginger, the tahini, the minced garlic, the lime/lemon juice, the tamari, the almond butter, and the coconut sugar in a blender.
3. Pour in a bit of water and blend until a thick sauce is created.
4. Finally, obtain a large mixing basin and combine the zucchini noodles with the sauce.

5. Garnish with a squeeze of lime/lemon juice and a sprig of coriander before serving.

Nutrition

- Calories in a serving: 229
- Fat: 6.2 g
- Saturated fat: 3.8 g
- Cholesterol: 5 milligrams
- Sodium: 785 milligrams
- Carbohydrates: 13.7 g
- Fiber: 6.2 g

QUINOA WITH SPINACH

Time required for preparation: 10 minutes.
Cooking time: 25 minutes.
Servings: 4

Ingredients:
- 1 cup of cooked quinoa
- 2 cups of finely chopped fresh spinach
- 1/2 cups of spring water
- 1 sweet potato thinly sliced
- 1 teaspoon of ground coriander powder
- 1 teaspoon of turmeric
- 1 tbsp. of ground cumin seeds
- 1/2 teaspoon of freshly grated ginger
- 2 garlic cloves, peeled and chopped
- 1 cup of finely chopped onion
- 2 tablespoons of extra-virgin olive oil
- 1 tablespoon of freshly squeezed lime juice
- A pinch of salt

Instructions:
1. Add the onion and the olive oil in to the pan and cook for 2 minutes.
2. Stir in the garlic, ginger, spices and quinoa and cook for 10 minutes.
3. Combine the spinach, sweet potatoes, and water and cook for another 10 minutes.
4. Put on plates and serve.

Nutrition

- Calories in a serving: 268
- Fat: 9.9 g
- Carbohydrates: 38.8 g
- Sugar content: 3.4 g
- Protein content: 7.6 g

VEGGIE SOUP

Preparation time: 1 hour and 20 minutes

Serving: 4 servings

Ingredients:
- 4 cups of Garbanzo Beans that have been cooked
- Quinoa or Spelled Pasta (around 4 cups) cooked
- 4 cups of mushrooms, finely chopped
- 3 plum tomatoes, peeled and sliced
- 1 zucchini, peeled and sliced
- 2 cups of butternut squash, finely chopped
- 1 cup of red bell peppers, finely chopped
- 1 red onion, peeled and chopped
- 2 teaspoons of salt
- Avocado oil (about 2 teaspoons)
- 2 teaspoons of Basil

Instructions:
1. Fill a big pot halfway with Spring Water and bring it to a boil over high heat.
2. Preparing all of the vegetables (chop or dice them).
3. Combine all ingredients (except the pasta) and seasonings in a large stockpot. Boil for about 30 minutes.
4. Stir in the pasta cooked 5 minutes before the soup is done.
5. Pour your Veggie Soup into a bowl and enjoy!

Tip

You may serve our Veggie Soup with Tortillas or Spelled Bread as a side dish.

Nutrition

- Calories in a serving: 210
- Fat: 6.4 g
- Saturated fat: 2.8 g
- Carbohydrates: 11.3 g
- Fiber: 3.5 g

SOUP WITH SOURSOP

Preparation time: 1 hour and 20 minutes

Serving: 4

Ingredients:
- 4–6 Soursop Leaves
- 2 cups of kale, finely chopped
- 1 cup of Quinoa
- 1 cup of chopped Chayote Squash
- 1 cup of red bell peppers, finely chopped
- 1 cup of finely diced Onions
- 1 cup of sliced Zucchini (optional)
- 1 cup of sliced Summer Squash (optional)
- 3 tablespoons of Onion Powder
- A pinch of Himalayan Pink Salt
- 1 tablespoon of freshly minced ginger
- 1 tbsp. of dried oregano leaves
- 1/4 cup of basil (or parsley)

Instructions:
1. Prepare all vegetables (chop or dice them).
2. Combine all of the ingredients and seasonings in a large pot. 8 cups of spring water should be added.
3. Cook the mixture for 30–40 minutes on medium heat after the mixture reaches a rolling boil.
4. Toss the soup into a bowl and serve.

Tips
- If you don't have or don't like Quinoa, you can substitute it with rice or homemade pasta.

- This recipe does not require Cayenne Powder if you are not a fan of spicy food.
- As an alternative to Tortillas, you can serve Sour soup with Herb Bread.

Nutrition
- Calories in a serving: 230
- Fat: 6.4 g
- Saturated fat: 2.8 g
- Carbohydrates: 11.3 g
- Fiber: 3.5 g

SOUP WITH MUSHROOMS

Preparation time: 3 hours and 20 minutes

Serving: 4

Ingredients:
- 3 cups of Portobello Mushrooms,
- 1 cup of Garbanzo Beans that have been cooked
- 2 cups of aquafaba (plant-based yoghurt)
- 1 cup of kale, finely chopped
- 2 plum tomatoes, peeled and sliced
- Red Bell Peppers (about 1/2 cup)
- Chopped butternut squash,
- Chopped (about 1/2 cup) red onions,
- Diced (about half a cup)
- 2 tablespoons of Himalayan Pink Salt
- 2 teaspoons of Onion Powder (optional)
- 1 teaspoon of Basil (optional)
- 1 teaspoon of oregano (optional)
- A pinch of ground ginger powder
- 2 tablespoons of Grapeseed Oil

Instructions:
1. Put all the ingredients in a saucepan and cook over low heat for 1 hour. Be sure to stir constantly during this time.
2. Let it cool and mix everything with an immersion blender.
3. Serve the mushroom soup in bowls and enjoy!

Tips

- If you don't have any prepared Aquafaba on hand, you can use 4 cups of Spring Water for it.
- You can skip the Cayenne Powder if you don't like spicy foods.
- To accompany the Mushroom Soup, you can serve it with Tortillas or Herb Bread.

Nutrition

- Calories in a serving: 240
- Fat: 2.4 g
- Saturated fat: 4.8 g
- Carbohydrates: 11.3 g
- Fiber: 3.5 g

SOUP WITH TOMATOES AND BEANS

Preparation time: 1 hour and 20 minutes

Serving: 4

Ingredients:
- 3 cups of Garbanzo Beans that have been cooked
- 1 Tomatillo, finely chopped
- 10 plum tomatoes, peeled and sliced
- Green Bell Pepper (1/2 cup)
- Half cup of finely chopped onions.
- 2 tablespoons of Himalayan Pink Salt
- 1 teaspoon of Basil
- 1 teaspoon of cayenne pepper powder
- 1/2 teaspoon of oregano leaves
- Achiote powder (1/2 teaspoon)
- Grapeseed Oil (about 2 tablespoons)
- 1 cup of spring water (optional)

Instructions:
1. Place the tomatillos, onions, bell peppers, grape seed oil and herbs in a large pot. Sauté vegetables for 4–5 minutes on medium heat, stirring occasionally.
2. In a large saucepan, combine the tomatoes, spices, Garbanzo Beans, and spring water.
3. Cook for approximately 1 hour on a low heat setting.
4. Add vegetables in a soup a couple of minutes before the soup is finished cooking.

5. Dish up your Spicy Tomato Bean Soup and enjoy it while it's hot!

Tips

- Add only 1/2 teaspoon of Cayenne pepper instead if you prefer it to be a little less hot.
- Depending on your preference, spicy Tomato Bean Soup can be served with Tortillas or Herb Bread.

Nutrition
- Calories in a serving: 210
- Fat: 6.4 g
- Saturated fat: 2.8 g
- Carbohydrates: 15.3 g
- Fiber: 3.5 g

GAZPACHO WITH CREAMY CUCUMBER

Preparation time: 15 minutes

serving: 2

Ingredients

- 2 cucumbers
- 1 ripe avocado
- 1 Key Lime,
- 2 handfuls of Basil,
- A pinch of Himalayan Pink Salt
- 2 cups of spring water
- 2 tablespoons of extra virgin olive oil

Instructions:

1. Peel the cucumber and remove any seeds that may be present. Cut the avocado into pieces.
2. Place all ingredients in a blender and purée until smooth. Add the salt.
3. Put the soup to cool in the refrigerator for around 10 minutes.
4. To finish, add basil leaves, oil and thinly sliced cucumber to the dish and garnish with them.
5. Take pleasure in your Creamy Cucumber Gazpacho!

Tips

The Creamy Cucumber Gazpacho goes well with Chickpea "Tofu" snack, available separately.

Nutrition

- Calories in a serving: 135
- Fat: 2.4 g
- Saturated fat: 2.4 g
- Carbohydrates: 11.3 g
- Fiber: 3.5 g

SOUP WITH CREAMED ASPARAGUS

Time required for preparation: 10 minutes

Cooking time: 30 minutes

Servings: 2

Ingredients:
- 2 lb. fresh asparagus trimmed off woody stems
- 1 lime zest and 2 tablespoons lime juice
- 1/4 ounces of coconut milk
- 1 teaspoon of dried thyme
- 1/2 tbsp. of dried oregano
- 1 cauliflower head, florets removed from the head
- 1 tablespoon of minced garlic
- 1 leek, thinly sliced
- 3 tablespoons of coconut oil
- A pinch of pink Himalayan sea salt

Instructions:
1. Boil the asparagus, leek and cauliflower in a large pot filled with water.
2. Heat the coconut oil in a large pot. Add the cooked vegetables, herbs and lime juice. Cook for 5 minutes, mixing frequently.
3. Turn off the heat and blend everything with an immersion blender.
4. Allow to cool and serve on plates garnished with the chopped lime slices.
5. Serve.

Nutrition

- Calories in a serving: 110
- Fat: 6.4 g
- Saturated fat: 2.8 g
- Carbohydrates: 11.3 g
- Fiber: 3.5 g

FRESH SALAD

Preparation time: 5 minutes

Servings: 2

Ingredients

- half a cucumber cut into slices
- 2 cups of watercress, torn into pieces
- 1 lime zest and 2 tablespoons lime juice
- 4 cutlery nuts into small pieces
- 4 fresh basil leaves
- 1/2 teaspoon of turmeric powder
- 2 tablespoons of extra-virgin olive oil
- A pinch of Himalayan Pink Salt

Instructions:

1. Combine the olive oil and key lime juice in a large salad bowl. Mix them thoroughly to ensure that they are well-combined.
2. Add the thinly sliced vegetables, walnuts, turmeric, lime zest, salt and herbs.
3. Make sure everything is thoroughly mixed.
4. Dish up and enjoy your quick and easy Fresh Salad!

Nutrition

- Calories in a serving: 92
- Fat: 2.4 g
- Saturated fat: 2.4 g
- Carbohydrates: 11.3 g
- Fiber: 6.5 g

SALAD DE ZUCCHINI ET DE SQUASH

Time required for cooking: 30 minutes plus 1 hour in the refrigerator

Servings: 4

Ingredients
- 2 cups of shredded Zucchini
- Squash (about 1/2 cup) shredded
- 1/2 cup of Brazil Nuts that have been soaked (overnight or at least 4 hours)
- 1/4 cup of Hempseed Milk
- Onion, roughly diced (about a quarter cup)
- A quarter teaspoon of finely chopped dates
- A pinch of Himalayan Pink Salt
- 2 teaspoons of lime juice
- 1/2 cup of Water

Instructions:
1. Put all the thinly sliced vegetables in a salad bowl.
2. In a blender, combine the dates, hempseed milk, Brazil nuts, lime juice, salt, and 1/2 cup of spring water. Blend until smooth.
3. Season the vegetables with the freshly blended emulsion.
4. Serve immediately.

Nutrition
- Calories in a serving: 110
- Fat: 2.6 g
- Saturated fat: 2.6 g
- Carbohydrates: 11.5 g

- Fiber: 3.5 g

MANGO SALAD

Preparation time: 15 minutes

Size of each serving: 2

Ingredients:

- 6 plum tomatoes
- 1/2 cup of mango chunks (diced)
- 1 tomatillo (tomatillos are a type of tomato).
- red onions (about half a cup diced)
- 1/4 cup of chopped Green Bell Peppers
- Cilantro leaves (about 1/2 cup)
- A pinch of Himalayan Pink Salt
- A pinch of onion powder
- 2 teaspoons of lime juice
- 2 tablespoons of extra virgin olive oil

Instructions:

1. Cut all the vegetables thin and put them in a salad bowl.
2. Add the mango, lime juice and seasonings
3. Enjoy your Quick Mango Salad!

Tip

- You may serve our Tortilla Chips

Nutritions:

- Calories in a serving: 110
- Fat: 1.4 g
- Saturated fat: 1.8 g
- Carbohydrates: 15.3 g
- Fiber: 2.5 g

SALAD DE CHICKPEAS

Time required for cooking: 20 minutes plus 30–60 minutes in the refrigerator

Serving: 4

Ingredients
- 2 cups of chickpeas that have been cooked
- Vegan Mayonnaise (about ½ cup)
- Red onions, roughly chopped (about 1/4 cup)
- 1/2 cup of chopped Green Bell Peppers
- 1 teaspoon of Dill
- A pinch of onion powder
- A pinch of Himalayan Pink Salt

Instructions:
1. In a large bowl, combine chickpeas and vegan mayonnaise. Mix.
2. Blend all remaining ingredients and pour them into the salad bowl with the chickpeas. Mix up.
3. Refrigerate it for 30–60 minutes before serving.
4. Toss the Chickpea Salad together and serve.

Nutrition
- Calories in a serving: 110
- Fat: 5.4 g
- Saturated fat: 1.8 g
- Carbohydrates: 11.3 g
- Fiber: 4.5 g

SALAD WITH "POTATOES"

Time required for cooking: 20 minutes plus 30 minutes in the refrigerator

Servings: 4

Ingredients

- 2 sweet potatoes
- 2 zucchini
- 1 carrot
- 1 cup of Brazil Nuts that have been soaked (overnight or at least 4 hours)
- 1/4 cup of sliced Green Bell Peppers
- ½ onion
- 1 tablespoon of lime juice
- Avocado Oil
- A pinch of Himalayan Pink Salt
- A pinch of Ginger Powder
- 1/2 cup of spring water
-

Instructions:

1. 1 In a blender, combine the Brazil Nuts, Avocado Oil, Lime Juice, spices, and 1/2 cup of   Spring Water until smooth. 1 minute of vigorous blending later, you have a smooth paste.
2. Boil carrot, sweet potatoes, zucchinis and onion: let them cool and cut them into slices.
3. Combine everything in a salad bowl and mix.
4. Allow 30 minutes of cooling time in the refrigerator before serving.
5. Plate your "Potato" Salad and enjoy it immediately!

Nutrition
- Calories in a serving: 274
- Fat: 5.4 g
- Saturated fat: 2.8 g
- Carbohydrates: 19.3 g
- Fiber: 4.5 g

PICKLE SALAD

Time required for cooking: 20 minutes plus 30 minutes in the refrigerator

Serving: 2

Ingredients:
- 1 cup of cucumbers, cut thinly
- 1/2 cup of lime juice,
- ½ cup of apple cider vinegar
- 1 tablespoon of fresh dill
- 1 teaspoon of coriander
- 1 teaspoon of Himalayan Pink Salt
- Red pepper crushed to taste (or a half teaspoon).
- 1/2 cup of Spring Water

Instructions:
1. Crush the coriander using a pestle and mortar.
2. Combine the cucumber slices, coriander, and the remaining ingredients in a jar with a tight-fitting cover. Shake it up thoroughly.
3. Allow it to infuse for 6–8 hours, shaking it every 1–2 hours during that time.
4. Serve your Pickle Salad and enjoy it.

Nutrition
- Calories in a serving: 110
- Fat: 2.4 g
- Saturated fat: 1.4g
- Carbohydrates: 16.3 g

- Fiber: 3.6 g

BEANS IN A BAKED TOMATO SAUCE

Preparation time: 1 hour and 40 minutes
Serving: 4
Ingredients:

- 6 plum tomatoes
- 3 cups of Garbanzo Beans that have been cooked
- 1/4 cup of sliced Green Bell Peppers
- Onion, diced (about 1/4 cup)
- 3 tablespoons of Date Syrup
- A pinch of Onion Powder
- A pinch of Himalayan Pink Salt
- A piece of freshly grated ginger
- a quarter teaspoon of turmeric powder
- 1/8 teaspoon of powder Cloves

Instructions:

1. Blend the Plum Tomatoes, Date Syrup and herbs until they have a smooth consistency in a blender.
2. Combine the tomato mixture, bell peppers, onions, and Garbanzo Beans in a large saucepan.
3. Cook, turning periodically, on medium heat for approximately 30 minutes, or until tender vegetables.
4. Serve.

Nutrition

- Calories in a serving: 110
- Fat: 6.4 g
- Saturated fat: 2.8 g
- Carbohydrates: 11.3 g
- Fiber: 3.5 g

LINKS OF SAUSAGE

Preparation time: 30 minutes
Serving: 4
Ingredients:

- Mushrooms, quartered (about 1 cup)
- 2 cups of Garbanzo Beans that have been cooked
- a half cup of finely chopped onion
- 4 fresh basil leaves
- 1 teaspoon of dill
- 1 tablespoon of onion powder
- A pinch of garlic powder
- 1 teaspoon of dried sage (ground)
- 1 teaspoon of oregano
- A pinch of Himalayan Pink Salt
- Avocado Oil (about 2 teaspoons)

Instructions:

1. Blend all ingredients (except avocado Oil and Garbanzo Bean) until smooth.
2. Add the Garbanzo Beans to the prepared mixture and blend for another 30 seconds, or until everything is thoroughly blended.
3. Make a stencil by filling a piping bag with the mixture and snipping off a small piece of the bottom corner.
4. Form sausages by squeezing the prepared mixture.
5. Heat the avocado Oil in a skillet over medium heat until hot.
6. Cook them for 3–4 minutes on each side, or until they are golden brown. They must be turned with care to avoid them breaking apart.
7. Serve with a fresh salad.

Advice

You can serve it with Sauce or Vegan Mayonnaise

Nutrition

- Calories in a serving: 476
- Fat: 5.4 g
- Saturated fat: 2.8 g
- Carbohydrates: 16.3 g
- Fiber: 3.5 g

DESSERTS

CHOCOLATE CREAM

Preparation time: 5 minutes
Serving: 2
Ingredients:

- 100 gr agave syrup
- 40 gr of cocoa powder
- 5 gr of vanilla powder
- 50 gr almond or soy milk
- a pinch of cinnamon

Instructions:

1. mix all ingredients except cinnamon vigorously.
2. Sprinkle cinnamon to taste.

You can add more milk and heat it up to obtain a delicious hot drink.

PUMPKIN TIRAMISU

Preparation time: 30 minutes
Serving: 4
Ingredients:

- 4 whole wheat spelt toasts or 4 dry spelt cookies
- 1 cup of pumpkin puree made by steaming pumpkin cut into pieces
- 2 tablespoons agave syrup
- 4 tablespoons of Soy Milk
- 2 cups of coffee
- Bitter cocoa

Instructions:

1. Blend the pumpkin with soy milk and agave syrup
2. Place the rusks on the bottom of a mug a -single portion.
3. Pour over the cups of coffee.
4. Cover with the pumpkin cream and level off well.
5. Sprinkle with unsweetened cocoa powder.

Origins of the recipe:

Tiramisu', wich means adds life, is a tipicle Italian dessert created in the mid-1800s in the city of Trevis. It seems that this dessert was created by a mistress of a pleasure house so she could offer it to her customers. She considered this dessert to be an aphrodisiac.

CHOCOLATE SALAMI

Preparation time: 30 minutes

Serving: 4

Ingredients:

- 300 grams of dark chocolate min 85 %.
- 150 grams of rice crackers
- 200 grams of soy milk
- 200 grams of dried fruit
- 1 teaspoon of cinnamon powder
- 1 teaspoon of turmeric powder

Instructions:

1. chop the galettes and the dried fruit together.
2. melt the chocolate in the microwave and let it cool off.
3. add the soy milk and the chopped biscuits and dried fruit.
4. mix well and pour everything on a sheet of baking paper.
5. wrap the baking paper into a cylinder and roll up the ends to close it.
6. Chill the roll in the fridge for at least 2 hours.
7. unroll and cut the chocolate salami into slices.

Deepening:

Typical Italian dessert prepared especially after the Easter holidays in order to reuse the leftover Easter egg chocolate.

CHOCOLATE CREAM AND BEANS

Preparation time: 30 minutes
Serving: 4

Ingredients:

- 400 grams of cooked black beans
- 1/2 cup of beloved cocoa
- 3 cups of almond milk
- a tablespoon of agave syrup
- one teaspoon of cinnamon powder
- crumbled dried fruit
- garnish with sliced strawberries

Preparation:

1. Place all ingredients in a large bowl and blend with an immersion blender
2. Divide the cream into 4 cups and chill them in the refrigerator for an hour.
3. Garnish with slices of strawberries.

This dessert has a low glycemic index.

CHOCOLATE AND YOGURT CAKE

Preparation time: 20 minutes

Serving: 4

Ingredients:

- 1 jar of vegetable yogurt 125 g
- 1 jar of sunflower oil
- 1/2 a jar of agave syrup
- 1 jar of almond or soy milk
- 1 jar of spelt flour
- 1 jar of rice flour
- 1 tablespoon of unsweetened cocoa
- 1 sachet of baking powder

Preparation:

1. Empty the yogurt jar into a large bowl.
2. Add all the other ingredients except for the cocoa and mix well until you get a creamy mixture.
3. Divide the dough into two bowls and in one add the bitter cocoa and stir well.
4. Line a cake tin with baking paper and pour the dough of the first bowl in it then pour the other cacao dough in the center of the cake tin.
5. Bake at 180 degrees for 25 minutes.

Additional information: this dessert is very easy to prepare because there is no need for scales!

14-DAY MEAL PLAN

All the recipes I proposed in this book can be used to compose your personalized meal plan.

Below I have prepared a 14-day meal plan that corresponds to an appropriate period for you to be able to achieve detoxification and activate an anti-inflammatory process in the body.

Feel free to modify some dishes with others suggested in my recipes that suit your tastes more.

Or if you are particularly in a hurry you can simplify the daily menu as follows:

- for breakfast, prepare a nutritious smoothy with unsweetened vegetable yogurt blended with fresh fruit, half an avocado and a handful of dried fruit

- at lunch you can opt for a simple spelled or quinoa salad with lots of fresh vegetables and a fruit

- you can dine with a tasty cereal and mushroom soup combined with a slice spelled bread topped with rosemary and olive oil

- the snack can be based on dried fruit or berries.

Please read the valuable rules I have prepared for you before reviewing the 14-Day Meal Plan. The rules will make your cooking time more efficient!

Rules

- Before beginning to prepare any meal you should carefully read the daily tips.
- The snacks are optional.
- You can customize your meal by including extras like salads made from fresh vegetables, sauces, fruits, pure agave syrup, tortillas, and so on.

Day 1

Breakfast: Smoothy with unsweetened vegetable yogurt blended with fresh fruit, half an avocado and agave syrup 4 brazil nuts, ginger tea.

Lunch: Mushroom Soup with Herb Bread lunch
                A fresh salad with ½ avocado

Dinner: Cabbage Roll Casserole with a Twist
                Zucchini and Squash Salad.

Snack: Smoothie with avocado and fresh fruit

Preparation Tips:

1. Make an extra batch of Mushroom Soup and keep it in the fridge for Day 2

2. Keep the remaining Herb Bread for Day 2 as a snack

Day 2

Breakfast: Strawberry Milkshake with vegetable milk

A handful of almonds

Lunch: Quinoa with Spinach

Dinner: Gazpacho with Creamy Cucumber
               A slice of spelled bread with olive oil

Snack: Strawberry Milkshake with vegetable milk

Preparation tips:

1. Make an additional portion of Quinoa and keep it in the refrigerator for Day 3

2. Buy two additional portions of spelled bread

Day 3

Breakfast: Alkaline Porridge with Fruits   A handful of walnuts

Lunch: Pizza with Basil and Olives
           Lettuce salad with sesame seeds

Dinner: Black bean chili
            Tomato and basil salad with olive oil

Snack: Tortilla Chips with a dipping sauce called "Cheese.
Preparation tips:

1. Prepare four extra portions of Black bean chili for Day 5 (look at dinner).

2. Prepare a second batch of Tortilla Chips for Day 4 as a backup plan (look at snack).

Day 4

Breakfast: Coconut Tahini Cookies made with permitted flours
A cup of coconut milk

Lunch: Quinoa Burrito Bowl
Thin cut raw courgettes with sesame seeds and avocado oil

Dinner: Pasta with Tomatoes and Spelt
A plate of spinach cooked with avocado oil

Snack: Tortilla Chips with Quick Mango Salsa
Preparation tips:

1. Make an additional batch of Pasta with Tomatoes and Spelt for Day 5 (look at dinner).

2. Preparing an extra portion of Quinoa Burrito Bowl for Day 6 is optional (look at lunch).

Day 5

Breakfast: Slice of fresh coconut
A cup of chamomile
A little banana

Lunch: Stir-Fry with Zucchini and Broccoli

Dinner: Pasta with Tomatoes and Spelt
Cucumber salad with slides of mushrooms and avocado oil

Snack: A handful of berries and nuts

Preparation tips:

Make an additional serving of broccoli in the fridge for Day 6. (look at lunch).

1. Preparing an extra portion of Pasta with Tomatoes and Spelt for Day 7 is recommended (look at dinner).

Day 6

Breakfast: Raspberry tea

A slice of spelled bread with thaini butter and

agave syrup

A handful of berries

Lunch: Salad de chickpeas
Broccoli with walnuts and sesame seeds oil

Dinner: Kamut Noodles with Pesto
Tomato and basil salad with olive oil

Snack: Strawberry Milkshake with vegetable milk

Preparation tips:

1. Keep an extra serving of Salad de chickpeas in the refrigerator for Day 8 (look at lunch).

2. Keep an extra serving Strawberry Milkshake with vegetable milk for breakfast

Day 7

Breakfast: Strawberry Milkshake with vegetable milk
A handful of walnuts

Lunch: Pasta with Tomatoes and Spelt
Zucchini and Squash Salad

Dinner: Links of Sausage
Broccoli with walnuts and sesame seeds oil

Snack: A handful of almonds

Preparation tips:

Make an extra batch of the Zucchini and Squash Salad or Day 8 (look at lunch).

Day 8

Breakfast: Coconut Tahini Cookies made with permitted flours

A cup of coconut milk

Lunch: Quinoa Burrito Bowl

            Thin cut raw courgettes with sesame seeds and

            avocado oil

Dinner: Zucchini and Squash Salad
            ½ avocado with a slides of tomato and olives

Snacks: Juice from Prickly Pears
Preparation tips:

Make an extra batch of Quinoa Burrito Bowl and keep it in the fridge for Day 10. (look at lunch).

Day 9

Breakfast: Pancakes with Strawberry Jam

Lunch: Okra with a Spicy Twist
            Thin cut raw courgettes with sesame seeds and
            avocado

Dinner: Chickpea Salad
            Lettuce salad with sesame seeds
Snack: Strawberry Milkshake with vegetable milk

Preparation tips:

1. Make an additional batch of Strawberry Milkshake with vegetable milk to use on Day 10 (look at snack).

2. Preserve an additional serving of Okra with a Spicy Twist for Day 10 (look at lunch).

Day 10

Breakfast: Strawberry Milkshake with vegetable milk
A handful of almonds

Lunch: Okra with a Spicy Twist
Broccoli with walnuts and sesame seeds oil

Dinner: Pizza with Basil and Olives

Lettuce salad with sesame seeds

Snack: A handful of berries and nuts

Preparation tips:

Day 11 will require an extra portion of Pizza with Basil and Olives (look at dinner).

Day 11

Breakfast: Raspberry tea

A slice of spelled bread with thaini butter and

agave syrup

Lunch: Pizza with Basil and Olives
              Lettuce salad with sesame seeds

Dinner: Zucchini and Squash Salad

              ½ avocado with slices of tomato and olives

Snack: Juice from Prickly Pears

Preparation tips:

Keep the leftover Zucchini and Squash Salad for Day 13 in an airtight container (look at dinner).

Day 12

Breakfast: Strawberry Milkshake with vegetable milk

              A handful of walnuts

Lunch: Pasta with Tomatoes and Spelt

              Zucchini and Squash Salad

Dinner: Links of Sausage

              Broccoli with walnuts and sesame seeds oil

Snack: A handful of almonds

Preparation tips:

Reserve a portion of the Pasta with Tomatoes and Spelt for Day 13 of the week (look at lunch).

Day 13

Breakfast: Tempeh with Pineapple on the Grill

Lunch: Salad de chickpeas

Broccoli with walnuts and sesame seeds oil

Dinner: Pasta with Tomatoes and Spelt
½ avocado with slices of tomato and olives

Snack: A handful of berries and nuts

Preparation tips:

Making additional Salad de chickpeas for Day 14 will save you time and money (look at lunch)

Day 14

Breakfast: Slice of fresh coconut

A cup of chamomile

A little banana
Lunch : Green Soup with Alkalizing Properties
Tomato and basil salad with olive oil
Dinner: Salad de chickpeas
Cucumber salad with slides of mushrooms and avocado oil

Snacks: A handful of berries and nuts

Made in the USA
Monee, IL
11 April 2022

94456525R00154